ANYTHING IS POSSIBLE

ANYTHING IS POSSIBLE

TURNING YOUR LIFE AROUND AFTER TRAUMA

JOSEPHINE MARIPOSA

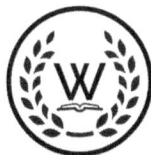

WINNERS
PRESS

Copyright © 2020 by Josephine Mariposa

Published in the United States by Winners Press, an imprint of Winners LLC, winnerspress.com.

ISBN: 978-0-9712240-4-9

Printed in the United States of America

Cover photography by Ben Meek

I have decided that I can't be the person I was, but I don't have to be a shadow of myself. I've chosen to find someone, somewhere in between, using the tools I have.

— Tina McDonald

CONTENTS

PREFACE

A Parable

A farmer went out to sow his seed. As he was
scattering the seed, some fell along the path,
and the birds came and ate it up. Some fell on
rocky places, where it did not have much soil. It
sprang up quickly because the soil was shallow.
But when the sun came up, the plants were
scorched, and they withered because they had
no root. Other seed fell among thorns, which
grew up and choked the plants. Still, other seed
fell on good soil, where it produced a crop—a
hundred, sixty or thirty times what was sown.
Whoever has ears, let them hear.

    — Matthew 13, Verses 1-9 and 18-23

I thought I had life figured out: a satisfying career, great family. Then from one moment to the next, I got slapped in the face and suffered a stroke. That was my first experience of a life-changing event. Over the next two years, I would lose more functions resulting in an incomplete yet devastating spinal cord injury.

We never accept the possibility that life can change in an instant. We imagine we have years of life as well as a bright future ahead. Most of the time we cannot or do not want to accept the possibility that life is fragile, and self-care needs to be a priority for our survival. We are busy.

Life-changing moments and tragedies seem to happen to other people. We carry on merrily every day as if we are invincible and unaffected by tragedy. We are aware of accidents or life-transforming illnesses that happen to other people and yet are incredulous and completely unprepared when it happens to us.

The reason for writing this book is to present the possibility that a physical trauma does not have to be the ending of life as you knew it. Instead, it simultaneously offers an opportunity for growth after trauma.

With this story, I want to encourage you to consider the possibility that a physical trauma is not an ending of your life. The shock has changed everything. But you can also begin to see it as the beginning of the next chapter of your life. Rather than staying stuck in a state of post-traumatic stress disorder (PTSD), I hope you will see it as a seed, exposed by the shock, that will cause you to continue to grow.

This book aims to describe the thoughts and actions I have used to turn my life around after trauma, living it at its optimum. I hope it will give you ideas and strategies that will help you turn your disability or challenge on its head. My wish for you is to find a way to become differently able. Above all, it's a story with an unexpected ending.

Perhaps the most fantastic germination process in nature is that some species require fire for their seeds to sprout. These fruits can only release their seeds after the heat of the fire has physically melted the resin that holds them. Some of these seeds will only sprout in the presence of chemicals released in a fire. These seeds can remain buried in the soil bank for decades until a wildfire awakens them.

As a mother, storyteller, early childhood practitioner, and counselor, I have experience in dealing with crisis management. This experience has prepared me to explore the processes we face

when life hits us for six,[1] out of the blue. At this
moment, you might think about how my words are
going to change your perspective. I don't know the
answer to that question; that must be your choice.
You may feel you have nothing else to lose
currently, but there is another option.

The aftermath of an accident can result in
post-traumatic stress growth (PTSG), a sibling of
the more familiar post-traumatic stress disorder.
The priority of the medical profession is to fix the
physical body. There is no time in the hospital to
guide an individual through the mental and
spiritual process to turn a traumatic event into an
opportunity for growth and development. My wish
is to sow the seeds for that possibility, and as
described in the parable mentioned above, the
outcome may well depend on where you think the
seeds fell.

INTRODUCTION

That which does not kill us makes us stronger.
— Friedrich Nietzsche.

Trauma is not necessarily an entirely negative thing, though it is typically viewed that way. Trauma can result from many events, not only of physical injury, but also divorce, bereavement, sexual assault, military combat, and terrorist attacks. According to social psychologist and global thought leader Jonathan Haidt, "Individuals with post-traumatic stress disorder (PTSD) find no benefit from their trauma, only pain and anxiety."[1]

Counselors historically saw stress and trauma through a negative lens with implications on patients' lives. Before naming post-traumatic stress growth (PTSG) as a possible psychological process, post-traumatic stress disorder and its negative consequences as a result of stressors were the only options.

What if as a result of a trauma you emerged feeling stronger, finding resources you never knew you had in you? Suppose it gave you the confidence to face anything knowing that if you survived this, you could survive anything? What if trauma served as the catalyst to strengthen your relationships, helping you to discover who your real friends and support network are in life? Your priorities and perspective for the moment change. You start living in the moment and prioritizing what is important to you, giving you a better angle on life. What if you continue living as your authentic self?

The natural process that fascinated me most as a child was the transformation of a caterpillar into a butterfly. Somehow something prompts the caterpillar to change. Chemical changes within its DNA suddenly inspire it to build a cocoon around itself made of silk threads. When that is complete, a chemical process dissolves the caterpillar. Using its imago, the embedded imprint of what it is to become, the cells that survive the meltdown create another physical body utterly different from the one the caterpillar once had. It develops and dissolves again until finally, it creates itself as a butterfly. The creature finds a way to haul itself through a tiny space out of the cocoon before it emerges and then takes flight. It is an arduous process that takes time. All the while it remains vulnerable, and should we try to help by cutting open the cocoon, the butterfly will die.

The blueprint, an imago, of what the caterpillar is going to be is inside. Within us, we too have a blueprint of who we are at a soul level, what our life purpose is, and what we are to become. God has a plan for us. Society may mould us into a caterpillar, and then something unexpected and traumatic happens in a flash, out of the blue. Our real personality and imago emerge and start creating an urge to form a cocoon into which we dissolve and reappear differently able.

Our true self did not find expression in the body we once had. A caterpillar will not fly. Throughout the process of transformation, the caterpillar—broken, dissolves and re-emerges as the butterfly. Whatever brought you to this moment, whatever your injury, trust the process. You too may re-emerge a stronger, more beautiful expression of your true self to shine your light upon the world. The caterpillar does not start its life thinking one day it is going to fly and does not understand how it will become a butterfly. But anything is possible.

Bad things happen, and what determines the outcome is your attitude and perspective on what happened. Expect the unexpected. We cannot change what happened. It does not, however, mean that we are incapable of improving our outcomes. It may take many years. It is not what happens to us that defines our results. It is our attitude and dedication to change that impacts how and whether we grow.

Trust in God's plan and trust in yourself. If there is a pulse, there is hope. We do not need to know the details of why we are here or what God's plan is for us. If we are alive, we have a purpose. Trust that God has a plan for you. "Yeah, right," I hear you say. I said the same. If you are ready to explore a different way, however improbable to you, read on. I will be with you accompanying you virtually on your journey. My journey and injury may be different from yours; however, the process of recovery could be similar. Are you ready? Great! Time to rest. See you in the next chapter. In the meantime, don't get stuck in the trauma!

1

THE MAIN EVENT

Your present circumstances don't determine
where you can go; they merely determine where
you start.
— Nido Quebein

Something monumental changed my life. It was
something unexpected, fearful, and tragic. Or so I
thought.

It was 2011, and my daughter was
accompanying me from the United Kingdom to
Belgium for my uncle's funeral. We travelled by
train as my daughter favoured public transport
and could join the train at the next station. The
journey was pleasant and an extraordinary
experience on the Eurostar. As we both practice

minimalism, we stayed in a converted nunnery in the city and prepared ourselves to meet the whole family for the rather sombre occasion. After a nourishing breakfast, we set off by train to the venue. It was a rather stoic occasion. It was also stifling hot with beautiful, albeit oppressing sunshine. We discussed how a funeral could lack emotion and agreed we both felt we witnessed a bizarre form of saying goodbye that day.

In the evening, my maternal aunt invited us for a homecooked meal. The differences between my culture at birth and my culture at the time offered a topic of lively conversation and comparison. After enjoying a nourishing meal with a glass of wine, we returned to our monastic bedroom rather late at night, tired but happy, having partaken in a family-focused day. Going to bed, we were utterly exhausted by it all.

I awoke at 4 a.m. to use the bathroom and sleepily watched myself in the mirror, as was my habit of doing. I smiled at myself and said hello, and somewhere in my awareness, I noticed my mouth looked a bit crooked. I staggered a bit but thought nothing of it due to the lack of sleep, having enjoyed the wine, and acting a bit uncoordinated the night before. I head back to bed.

Upon waking, as I was still so tired, I suggested we take the day slowly. Having all day to travel back, we took each step deliberately. Breakfast was awkward, and I was unable to walk to the buffet table with ease, but my daughter helped bring things to the table. I drooled and was embarrassed, yet felt it was essential to eat before the long journey home ahead of us. When it came to paying the bill, I could not remember my PIN, but as the hotel had used my credit card for the deposit, we managed to complete that transaction.

We sauntered to the tram[1] stop. The tram would take us to the next step in our journey, the train station. Suddenly, I was no longer able to slot the coins in the meter and needed assistance to complete that small task. I was confused but got onto the tram and sat down quietly. What was going on? Did I have a hangover?

I reflected on how difficult things were that day, utterly oblivious to my surroundings. Arriving at the central train station to take the Eurostar, things got trickier. I wondered how on earth I was going to manage to push my ticket through the barrier, take my luggage, and show my passport at the same time. Multitasking was no longer possible. I followed my daughter like a drunk puppy, and how we got through customs is still a mystery.

I tried to tell my daughter that things were challenging to do. She stood up to ask the receptionist at the Eurostar desk whether we could rearrange our seats nearer, but they could not do that. As an alternative, they suggested we could have priority boarding, which meant we would have more time to board the train and enter the train as soon as possible. My brain had got into what I can only describe as la-la land. I could function to a certain degree, was very relaxed, and behaved as if entirely under the influence. I was, therefore, not fearful nor unhappy, just a bit confused.

My daughter bought me a cheese baguette for lunch, and it took me ages to eat, forty-five minutes to be exact. It seemed reasonable that day. She, however, was growing more and more concerned. I could read her facial expression but had no idea why she looked so thoughtful. After all, it was just a journey on the train.

Back in London, she asked me to sit in the waiting area and not walk off. She had to check something out. When she returned, she admitted she was looking for the NHS walk-in surgery. Still, being Sunday, it was not operational. I remember arguing why she thought I needed that service and that I had no intention to stay in London and the subject closed.

As we walked towards the train, I suddenly felt drunk and found it difficult to talk. Only a chatter came out. On the train home, my daughter did her best to appear calm.

"Sleep, Mum. We will soon be there."

So I closed my eyes and drifted off. Little did I know that she was ringing her brothers for help, but all three were playing a cricket match away and were not at home. She had to phone her dad, although she had not wanted to worry him. She asked him to come and collect me from the station and take me to the emergency room. The next obstacle was to overcome how to supervise me because her ticket was not valid for the entire journey.

She managed to strike up a conversation with a young family who assured her they would help me off the train onto the platform where her dad would be waiting.

"Promise me, Mum, you will go straight to the emergency room." In la-la land, I had not a care in the world. "You will tell them what has happened, won't you?" but I only looked confused. Then she started scribbling a note with all my information and contact numbers and putting it in my jacket pocket. I felt like Paddington bear, who stood on the platform of Paddington Station with a sign saying, "please look after this bear." She left at the next station and left me in the care of a young couple. I sat quietly in the corner, not saying much. When we reached the station, I spotted my husband on another platform. The young couple were true to their word and helped me off the train, settling me on a bench while I spied my husband running and arriving short of breath.

Helped out of the train and sitting on the bench, he assisted me and told me categorically not to talk. In the car, he drove me to the hospital. Sitting in the car, wondering why we were at the hospital with the note stuck to my coat. Two nurses came with a wheelchair. They took one look at the summary and rushed me straight to the ER. I had some experience with emergency rooms, having taken my children there on numerous occasions. We often had to wait for hours while the medical staff looked after those needing vital emergency care first. Even in la-la land, I registered that something vitally important and dangerous had happened, but what?

After two scans, it was confirmed that I had suffered a stroke. My brain was so muddled, I spoke to the nurse in Flemish, my language of origin, and wondered why she did not understand me. Two days later, I managed to speak English with a French accent. My husband agreed that he could live with it. We had enjoyed an English television series set in wartime France where the main characters spoke in this way. A few weeks later, however, my speech would return to normal.

Lifting a spoon to my mouth was painful. I could only eat with my non-dominant left hand. Walking with a nearly paralyzed right side was challenging. I am nothing but persevering in character. So that's what I did, moan and persevere.

The day following my arrival in the ER, the most meaningful words uttered to me by the physiotherapist were to imagine there had been a crash on the motorway. There was a lot of debris, but the road was still there. I would have to take another route to get to my destination, and it might take me longer to get there. By explaining what had happened this way, the physiotherapist described the cerebral event in a way I could understand even though my brain was injured. The clever explanation was not only helpful to accept what had happened, but it provided a solution as to how change could be effected. It was an effective metaphor I could absorb.

They moved me to a rehab hospital after three days. I had to learn to walk all over again, except now I was using a painful, heavy, useless right leg. The whole time in the hospital, I was dazed and not present. I seemed to see everything in slow motion. Thankfully, the nursing staff was patient, cared well for me, and was very understanding.

After three months, I was going home, and of all things, my test for release was being able to use the toaster and successfully make a cup of tea. How was I going to prepare meals for a family of five? I had no idea, but at least I had passed the examination. After I went home, I was sitting in the chair with the remote, and my son came in asking me what was for dinner. I told him I was going to ask him the same question, and we both realized we had to work together as a team.

Visits from the physiotherapist followed daily. There were many experiences in my life that had created neural pathways. Although I did not initially recognize why the physiotherapist wanted me to play the piano again, I misplayed it with the right hand. I came to understand that I had created vast neural pathways learning to play the piano. By reactivating them, my brain was able to reconnect some damaged ones. Currently, I can use my right hand, but it is much weaker than the left.

Six months later, I collapsed in the bathroom in a miserable place. If you live with four men, you know what I mean. My oldest son, whose bedroom was closest, came to see what the noise was all about, and seeing me lying there, he whispered and said he would get his father. My husband took one look at me and called an ambulance. The first responder came, and off we went to the emergency room again.

It was a bit like déjà vu: lots of tests, and back in the stroke ward. But I had managed it once, so I knew what to expect. However, this time, the scans did not confirm I had suffered another stroke but showed a lesion[2] in my neck. Because of that, I was transferred to a side room, an extension of the stroke ward, while they decided on the next step.

The examinations seemed endless. A registrar[3] from the Neurology department visited and was very insistent that her consultant neurologist come and evaluate me. I later found out the consultant was due to leave for his annual holiday. The last thing he probably expected was to visit a patient who had been diagnosed with a mysterious lesion in her neck.

He did a neurology examination followed by lots of furrowed brows. Judging by his next question, it appeared he had equally furrowed thinking.

"What has happened?"

I thought the man was somewhat lost in his head. He was the doctor! It seemed I should have been the one asking him that question, but I went along with it and did the best I could to answer. I informed him of the random functions in my body that were breaking down or having difficulty functioning. I also made him aware of the various departments I had visited relating to those losses of functions. Having exhausted the extent of my medical knowledge, I reverted to patient mode.

"I don't know what to expect next or what is going on," I told him. "I lack the medical knowledge to help myself. I have tried to eat clean, reduce stress, but nothing seems to stop these irregularities from happening."

He nodded slightly, followed by more frowning and raised eyebrows. I couldn't tell if he was in deep thought or just plain bored with my explanation.

"Okay," he said, "we will transfer you to neurology as soon as a bed is available."

His requests for tests were followed by a

barrage of demands to the registrar who was nodding as quickly as she was writing them down. The neurologist, not willing to take any additional time away from his holiday plans, could not leave the room fast enough. Meanwhile, I remained in the side room, waiting for a bed to be vacated in the neurology ward adjacent. I was neither a stroke patient nor a neurology patient. I was in limbo.

Judging by the number of blood tests I had to submit, I was sure a vampire was in charge of the phlebotomy lab. Next came the first of many lumbar punctures, aka spinal taps, a medical procedure in which they remove some spinal fluid that helps to diagnose diseases of the central nervous system. There would be nine in total before it was all said and done. I was just trying to get through this first one. The thought of a gigantic needle being inserted into my spine was enough to reduce me to tears. I phoned my older son, who wanted to be a doctor.

"I am scared. It's so invasive." I said, crying down the phone.

The sound of his crying mother must not have been much of a confidence-booster for him. Still, he was so calm.

"Mum, you have to let them do it because it's

the only way for them to find out what is making you ill. Without it, whatever it is will get worse."

Faced with that answer, he had suddenly become an 18-year-old voice of reason.

I was frantically trying to figure out how I was going to prepare myself for the lumbar puncture. I was terrified on the one hand, but on the other hand, it was clear it was essential. The registrar, a young lady wearing heels that clicked when she walked, announced she would be back the next morning to carry out the spinal tap. The thought of it was excruciating. But knowing it would last no longer than thirty minutes, I mentally prepared myself for what I imagined would be nothing less than a form of torture.

It's incredible what tricks our brains can play in building up an image of horror. The clicking of the heels down the corridor the next morning was just the right sound effects to frighten me again. The registrar entered the room with a trolley and matter-of-factly explained the procedure and what she expected of me. I tried to relax and accept that the next thirty minutes were going to be unpleasant, and they were. I prayed and prayed to just get through it.

"Okay, I have the sample."

Finally! She then put everything back on her

trolley and walked away, clicking her heels as she went. This time, I couldn't help but chuckle at the sound. It reminded me of a scene out of a James Bond movie of a Russian correctional officer. At least my imagination and sense of humour were still working in the background. Yes, the spinal tap had been unpleasant, but I only had to do it once, or so I thought. For now, it was over.

I was transferred to the neurology ward two weeks later as soon as a bed became available. Having not seen the doctor again for a while, I wondered what was next. I was upset and frustrated because nothing was happening.

One day, while my husband was visiting, the doctor appeared with an announcement.

"It's multiple sclerosis."

His delivery, which was as blunt as a hammer, matched his bedside manner. And the impact of his words hit me with just as much force. Multiple sclerosis (MS) is a condition that can affect the brain and the spinal cord and cause a wide range of symptoms. Some of these were identical to mine: blurred vision, loss of sensation, lack of movement in my legs, difficulties with balance, etc. I had looked after a lady who had been bedridden with MS and was very sad.

As tears filled my eyes, my husband took my

hand. "Whatever it is, remember you do not have to do this on your own. We are in this together."

This tender and loving moment made me cry even more. It reminded me of those desperate emotional scenes in movies. *I'm not in a film*, I told myself. *This is real. Get a grip.*

We talked through the night about the prospect of life with MS until we came to a degree of acceptance. The following morning, the doctor barged in.

"I was wrong. It's not MS. It's like MS, but you are too old for MS."

Not only had he thrown me back into the unknown, but he also called me old. I seriously thought he had an attitude.

Later on, I told my son about it as I was still quite a bit bothered. "Son, you're not likely to become a neurologist consultant."

"Why is that?"

"Because that man is rude, off the cuff, and dares to call me too old for some disease pattern. I am not nearer to knowing what this is even though I underwent that lumbar puncture." I could feel the heat rising in my face.

My son did his best to diffuse the situation. "Don't worry. They will find out what's happening. I have every confidence."

I was having a full-blown tantrum. It lasted a full hour and left me so exhausted that I slept for twelve hours. *Now what?*

The following morning, the phlebotomist came into the ward with her trolley announcing she needed more blood from me. Although she was very efficient, she took nine little vials of my blood, which seemed a bit excessive.

"Nine? Wasn't bloodletting a cure in the Middle Ages?"

She laughed, explaining they would do some more blood work and were keeping an eye on things.

"I am not likely to get out of here soon," I told my husband later. "Tests and more tests. I am getting used to being here now. Might as well submit."

He looked at me sideways with a comical expression. "Submit? That will be a first."

We both laughed. I certainly had been the most organized, determined, and career-focused woman in the past. My job had been in financial services initially. I studied early childhood education and was a practicing counselor. I also headed a charity working with families in crisis.

"You got this," he kept saying. I was not so sure about that. My body was telling me otherwise:

fevers, tremors, upset digestion daily, throwing up regularly, seeing double, and sleeping most of the day. I thought being asleep would at least get me through the day quicker. My mind was swimming with questions. Where do I start with all of this? How much longer before they would offer me a solution? What lay ahead, and how was I going to organize my life without losing the will to live?

2

STRENGTHENING THE THINGS WHICH REMAIN

Darkness deserves gratitude. It is the alleluia
point at which we learn to understand that all
growth does not take place in the sunlight.
  – Joan Chittister

Little did I know that the hospital ward would be
my home for the next two years. It felt like
returning to my childhood where needs are taken
care of by others. You have little opportunity to
express your individuality. My days were no longer
my own. It was like being assimilated by the Borg
from Star Trek. I was forced into the collective
mind of the institution, following the hospital's
methods instead of being independent and doing
what I wanted.

The daily routine ran with the precision of a military prison. Mornings started at the crack of dawn with vital statistics checks. Staff would then change, and there would be a medication round. Breakfast would be served in bed, followed by a bed wash, clothes change, and more doctor rounds. The never-ending tests, blood checks, and scans, were interrupted only by the lunchtime hour. Afternoons were slightly more relaxed with an enforced nap, some visiting, then winding down for the day. Even when I was asleep, vital checks would come around every four hours and wake me out of much-needed slumber.

I was a rebel as a child, and compliance was not my strongest suit. But here I had no choice but to submit. After a while, the routine became so embedded in my psyche, I would raise my left arm out from under the bedcovers and hand it over to the nursing staff for the blood pressure cuff without them even asking. I opened my mouth instinctively to enable them to take my temperature. Puke bowls became a constant fixture on my little bed table. As a mother of four children, I had had my fair share of morning sickness, and this was no different. Telling myself it would pass was a mechanism I used to deal with the daily bouts of nausea.

One day morphed into the next as I watched through bloodshot eyes and heavy eyelids each twenty-four hours fly by. I was no longer doing the usual things but gradually being returned to the state of a human being, resting when I could, and trying to find balance in my day. The highlight of each day was hoping I had no new symptoms, and I kept myself entertained by guessing what they would give me to eat next.

Eating has always been an essential pleasure to me, along with the joy of preparing meals. Hospital stays generally are short, so the menu would be the same every two weeks. There were options, of course, but I memorized the menu so well I could make my choices without even looking at it.

Those days, weeks, months, and ultimately years in the hospital were dark times. Week after week, there would be more tests, some more bizarre and memorable than others. I had plenty of time to reflect and ponder on how I could fill my time in between those endless tests. Thank goodness the blood in our bodies gets replenished, or I'm sure they would have drained me dry. It seemed every other day they would draw more blood to analyze. That was the best way to establish how my body processed food

and to determine which organs worked or
did not.

Every test came back negative, and I wondered
whether they would ever find the cause of me
being unwell. "Trust the process," my son kept
telling me. After the first year, I was beginning to
be impatient. I started behaving like a very
frustrated child. One night while my daughter was
visiting, I erupted in a flood of complaints. She
looked me in the eye, and in a voice barely over a
whisper she said, "Face it, Mum. You have never fit
in a box, and you are not going to now. You'll just
have to go with the flow." She was right. To get
treatment, I would require a diagnosis, and like it
or not, that meant continued testing.

Thinking was one of the few things my body
would still allow me to do independently, and my
mind was overrun with thoughts, all competing
for attention. I spent much time thinking about
why they call us human beings, yet we are so busy
filling our days doing things. It seemed to me,
"human doings" would best capture what we are. I
was glad to still be alive, and amidst the chaos, I
decided to go back to basics.

Being alive meant I was breathing, and
although I had heard of meditation, I had been far
too busy to give ten minutes a day to that in my

working life. Lying there, I started by paying attention to my breath and letting go of the myriad of thoughts zooming on inside my head. Having been a manager in charge of significant decisions, I had to accept that at that moment, I was not in control of anything. It felt like I was on the verge of an epiphany. Although I could not change anything outside my body, I could turn to the inside and start a conversation. Was that even possible?

Since I was already being awakened at dark-early hours anyway, I decided to begin a practice of meditation for ten minutes before the day would start in earnest. Having found a couple of apps on the phone, I would give myself time to evaluate them and practice breathing and meditation.

Being used to analyzing data in my jobs, I turned my attention to myself, my inner being. Quite often, when we lose control outside our comfort zone, we end up trying to control our environment. In my case, that consisted of a tiny bedside table with limited objects: my phone (a minicomputer really), a few get-well cards, and the dirty dishes left from whatever meal had just passed my lips. And let's not forget the ever-present accessory: a kidney-shaped sick bowl for when the meal on its way down decided to make its way back up. But first and foremost, I was alive and needed two things for that to continue: breathing and nutrients (food and water). Much of what was happening in my life was out of my control. But I decided to use what I could control to my best advantage.

If you do what you have always done, you will get the same outcome. Conversely, to get a different result, you must do something different. I started exploring meditation and breathing, listening through headphones. I thought I must be doing this wrong because not much seemed different. Immediate gratification is in abundance, but that is a principle that changes with a yearning for patience. Surely if millions of people paid attention to breathing and meditation, there had to be something to it.

Being a lifelong learner, meditation would give me a daily ritual and practice to do, as well as hopefully calming down the anxiety, stress, and feeling of being useless—worth giving it a go. I reminded myself that to get a different outcome, I had to try something different. I could measure how it affected me, if at all, by making a mental note of changes in my vital statistics, which, after all, were taken every four hours.

At the end of this book, I have shared resources that you may find useful that were available to me during my time in the hospital. Still, I encourage you to explore what apps are available and find one that works as a companion to aid you in breathing and meditation. The apps I used were free at that time. Currently, they ask for a subscription, but there are free videos on YouTube. One such video is by Eckhart Tolle, the author of *The Power of Now*, which is entertaining as well as informative and introduced me to the concept of "I am." Knowing that you are and understanding, "I am here" keeps your mind from residing in the past and remembering the things you used to be capable of doing. The past is just that, past. The intentional awareness of being present in the "I am" moment acts to prevent reliving the nightmare and the circumstances of your injury. At the same time, it stops you from panicking about the future and the uncertainty of "what if."

Being in the moment is a different way of being from the norm, which I found to be beneficial. Whenever thoughts would stray into the past or the future, I would silently say "thinking," but pay no attention to the thought. It became a sort of mind game.

Breathing is an unconscious action. Even if our bodies suffer high stress, the fact we are breathing is the first essential function of life. A baby being born and exiting its mother's womb would not survive long until it takes its first breath and fills its lungs with air. Let us live and learn to breathe while gaining as much benefit from that breath as we can.

The function of the respiratory system is to deliver air to the lungs. The lungs provide oxygen throughout the body via the blood. In contrast, carbon dioxide diffuses in the opposite direction. Out of the blood and into the lungs, out of our bodies via the out-breath.

When you're hospitalized or under related care, oxygen intake is one of those vital statistics monitored every four hours. You can evaluate your progress by checking the figure on the monitor. My lowest was 72 percent, but over time I could see it rise. Currently, it stays at over 90 percent, which is the best I can do with that resource. Knowing what that figure is will give you data as to how your body is processing vital oxygen. Watching the figures can be addictive as well as cause anxiety. I want you to let that go and just deep breathe regularly for ten minutes each day and see what happens.

As a next step, I tried yoga nidra. Yoga nidra or yogic sleep is a state of consciousness between waking and sleeping, like the "going-to-sleep" stage. It's typically induced by guided meditation, the next step after the introduction of breathing and meditation. The best time for me to practice this was during my afternoon nap. Invariably it sends you to sleep, relaxed yet focused on your body and inner being. Doing these three practices daily—breathing, meditation, and yoga nidra— not only helped to pass the time, but I also found my rhythm in between the hospital schedule.

Even though I still wasn't any closer to a diagnosis after the first six months, the breathing work helped me stay in the moment. A resident doctor, whose task is to look after the patients while the consultant is elsewhere, was visiting daily to update me. Still, the doctors and lab technicians found nothing. In those moments, it feels surreal, like you are imagining it all. Thankfully, the young doctor had not picked up the same bedside manner as the senior consultant. This one was nice to talk to and reminded me of my sons at home. He was in the process of buying a house, so we often talked about that. I could walk him through that process, which made me feel a bit useful, and as his house purchase grew closer, I shared his excitement.

One day he sat down on the chair next to me. He was smiling as usual, but there was a note of concern in his voice.

"They've found something, but it is highly unlikely that it is what it looks like it might be."

I was curious to know more after all these months of testing. "What is it?"

"The only person known with this caught it in an aircraft hangar. The source was traced to the material in his parachute. We can dismiss that because you don't have a connection with air hangars and parachutes."

Was I going to respond to that? Yes, of course, I was. "Maybe not directly, that is correct. But I do have a connection to silk."

"How?"

"I was a hand spinner." I had to share the information just in case.

"I don't think that will make a difference, but I will flag it."

The "what if" thoughts reared their ugly heads, but I was able to quell them with more meditation and yoga nidra.

A few days later, the conversation continued.

"They redid the test, but it was negative this time."

Another dead end. Part of me wanted a diagnosis because I was tired of being in limbo. Without a diagnosis, there is no medication to help, no equipment to assist in daily life, and the only possibility is to continue to rest. Resting is the way our body knows to reset.

Sleep plays an essential role in the function of the brain by forming new pathways and processing information. Research has shown that adequate sleep helps to improve memory and learning, increase attention and creativity, and aids in making decisions. What's not to love about sleep? The fact I slept more than my usual eight hours was an indicator of the level of rest my body needed to cope with whatever was happening.

A few weeks later, the consultant advised me that he had run out of options and was going to consult with the professor of neurology. His practice was about fifty miles away. However, the consultant told me that all consultants in the area met every other Wednesday to discuss cases, share resources, and share their knowledge.

"That's a good idea," I said. "I do a similar exercise with my children when we cannot find a solution to a problem. It amazes me the stuff they come up with that changes the perspective."

The days crawled by as I watched the calendar in anticipation of the consultants' meeting. *Patience*, I told myself. The blood work and regular vital checks continued, and it became my new routine. All the while I kept up with my breathing, meditation, and yoga nidra daily.

In preparation for the visit to the consultation with the professor of neurology, I felt in limbo. They discussed moving me to a cottage hospital[1] where they would continue to monitor me until they could get me an appointment at the teaching hospital. I had been to the cottage hospital previously to rehabilitate from my stroke, so I was able to envisage a more relaxed atmosphere since patients were mostly recovering or adapting to their new health situation. What I could not envision was what would happen next.

3

THE NEEDLE IN THE HAYSTACK

Call it a clan, call it a network, call it a tribe, call
it a family. Whatever you call it, whoever you
are, you need one.
— Jane Howard

As I was being transferred to a bed from the
stretcher, I noticed my physical body was not
interpreting feedback signals as usual. The
connections between my brain and body were not
in sync. It was as though a movement would cause
my brain to stammer, "Wh-Wh-What is h-h-
happening?"

Four people were rolling me from the stretcher
to the bed, and I panicked at the thought of falling
off the trolley. It was like the feeling you get when

you're falling in a dream, but you're lying still on the bed. My brain seemed to sometimes act independently of my body, sending signals that didn't fully make sense. I had to learn to quieten the mismatched signs and yet acknowledge them too. I found I was starting conversations with myself, even arguing. *I am finally losing it.*

The cottage hospital offered many advantages. I thought of it as a beautiful soft cocoon offering protection. Instead of staring at a brick wall as I did at the hospital, I now had a garden view. The colours, the sounds, and the visual stimulation of always seeing a different picture were the perfect escape from the four walls and my uncooperative body. Rain one day, sunshine the next, sunrises and sunsets, men working and maintaining the garden.

We do not think much about the nuances in the weather, but in those moments, every aspect of the garden was unique. I felt myself getting closer to God's creation. Sometimes there would be tracks from wildlife walking through the garden, and other days it would be the picture of serenity. Nature was a vision in which I could lose myself. It's so beneficial to reconnect with nature; it has such a therapeutic effect. In more contemplative moments, I wondered if that had anything to do with why we bring flowers to patients in the hospital. Is it to remind us of a connection to God's creation which we also are a part of, however we look or function?

They cared for me as you care for an infant. I was delicate and volatile. They washed me, dressed me, and fed me, all the while collecting data as to how my body was doing. I never dreamed that having a bath would become the highlight of my week. I looked forward to it more than an overworked employee looked forward to a two-week holiday. They would roll me into the bathroom on my bed, and they would hoist me into a protected strapped seat in the tub. There would be bubbles of my choice. A hair wash was heavenly, and I felt as if I was experiencing a spa session. After that, I would sleep for hours.

I had a lot more visitors than before. I had a daily visit from my husband and friends too. All the people that used to visit me in our shop missed me and kept coming to update me on what was happening in their lives. I felt like a celebrity. That was nice for my ego but terrible for my energy management. I just did not have the energy for everything. The nurses promised visitors would be screened and only allow those I felt capable of seeing. I felt like a bona fide diva.

My youngest son had a school lesson about the lady-in-waiting, someone who assists the queen with her daily activities. When he came for a visit later that day, he asked if I was a lady in waiting. I explained to him the difference between a lady in waiting and a lady who is just waiting. It was a kind thought from him, which touched my heart.

I missed my boys terribly. Yet it comforted me that even though I was away from them, I continued to be a central part of their lives. When my son phoned because he could not find his sports socks, I was able to help him find them. A visitor commented on how lovely it was to see the mum in me spring into action when needed despite how ill I looked. No matter how severe or debilitating the trauma, it doesn't stop you from being you.

For months I had been happy with my phone as entertainment. Suddenly, I lost functions and pressure in my hand. As a result, nothing would work. I said nothing, but my daughter started to notice lots of typing mistakes in my messages. This new health challenge was a further setback, and every time I used the phone, it would be a reminder of what I could no longer do. I felt like I'd lost a close friend, accompanied by a feeling of uncertainty. I wondered if this was a temporary loss or, worse yet, a permanent loss of function to overcome. *Would I ever get better? Was my life over?*

One afternoon I had a surprise visit from my oldest son and daughter. They had bought me an iPad with their own money as they saw it as an enhancement to my technological issues. When I am unable to do something, there is usually a piece of technology available to alleviate or remove the problem. An iPad offered a bigger screen, a Wi-Fi connection to access the internet, and a stylus pen to touch the screen. It put me in the mind of Maslow's hierarchy of needs. In addition to the basic physiological needs of shelter, food, and warmth, I think we need to add another layer. Wi-Fi has become another essential need to communicate and entertain.

My children's thoughtfulness to find a more adaptable solution to alleviate my frustration gave me an intense feeling of being loved. They saw solutions where I only saw deterioration or disappointment. Not only was I being cared for by medical staff, but my children were also showing me how much they loved me. It was a priceless feeling despite being out of sorts. I felt secure, loved, and comforted. Support between family members works both ways, although as a parent, that had never occurred to me. That was a big learning curve for me that day.

My youngest son told me I was just like the brain in an episode of *Futurama*.[1]

"Don't worry about your body, Mum. They can disconnect your body, attach you to a life-giving system, and you will still be able to function."

The solution to him seemed utterly plausible and straightforward. The enthusiasm of youth, I thought, all the while googling the contents of *Futurama* on my phone. The children were also adapting and drawing on the resources they had available. I was grateful for the existence of a cartoon that would ease my son's mind a little and provide some comfort.

A few weeks later, an appointment was scheduled for me to see the professor of neurology. At last! It would be a logistical exercise to get me there by ambulance on a stretcher accompanied by a healthcare assistant. I wondered if I would have the energy and presence of mind to absorb it.

The Prof. was concerned, deep in thought, not dissimilar to the first consultant whom I had thought distant. *Maybe they all act that way in Neurology*. There he sat unmoved, faced by an unwell woman who was emotionally distraught and could not stop crying. I had to believe he would be smart enough to solve this puzzle and trusted he was. The silence I had interpreted as detachment was, in fact, knowledgeable medics racking their brains to help find out what was happening to me. They were looking for the needle in the haystack. They were not giving up either, and I continued to believe they would find a diagnosis and treatment.

The journey there and back was exhausting, and the most I had to go on was that Prof. said he would be in touch. *In touch*, I thought, *what does that mean?* I continued crying and despairing, being in my emotional energy centre instead of my rational centre of thought.

Being in my emotional centre would become an indicator of lower energy levels, which affected my ability to process the medical information provided rationally. Sleep, I discovered, was the best solution.

After a few days back at the cottage hospital, I was still recovering from the trip away. I spent my days using the same effective self-care of breathing, meditation, and yoga nidra. There was no direct mention of the next step. But as the healthcare assistant took my lunch choice, she remarked that it would not really matter what I chose as I may be picked up by ambulance before lunch was served. Her slip of the tongue provided a hint. I was to be moved back to the medical ward. There, I would soon become the unwitting recipient of an extreme makeover of the medical kind.

4

TRANSITIONS

Not everything that is faced can be changed, but
nothing can be changed until it is faced.
— James Baldwin

The hospital schedule was hectic, so tests were
done wherever they could fit them in. Prof. had
ordered several different tests that would provide
data as to where the body was malfunctioning. I
got into the habit of expecting the unexpected, all
the while trying to keep my physical body stable,
meditate, and breathe. Praying and having
spiritual conversations were exciting moments too.
I reverted to saying my prayers at night. I would
eventually progress to listening for a response just
in case there was one. It was a soul-opening

experience. I got to understand myself on different levels and listen to the way my physical body was remaining stable and sometimes finding ways to heal something that was malfunctioning.

I turned my attention to nutrition and hydration. It seemed that whenever I felt confused and out of control, I would tidy up my hospital table and try to take pleasure in my food. At the teaching hospital where I was before, the diet was more varied, and I questioned why this hospital was so different. I discovered that the menu represents the food choices of the average population of patients. My area consisted mostly of seniors, and the menu of easy to chew foods and nursery puddings reflected that. In the teaching hospital, the average patient was more ethnically varied; hence, a different variety of options were available: stir-fries, curries, Caribbean dishes, etc.

The hospital menu, although adequate, was becoming a bit boring. I knew the choices without looking and frankly needed a little bit of a change. But it was the essential nutrition I needed, and it would have to do. However, it was worth asking if there were alternatives. I questioned the nurses who told me there was a special menu from which I could order. Full of joy, I ordered a baked potato with cheese and side salad. It was a simple adjustment, but it taught me two valuable lessons that made a big difference in this new world I was in. If you don't like the menu choices, it's worth exploring if the hospital provides different dietary options. Also, being able to make choices had shifted my entire perspective on the situation. A definite gain on the independence of thoughts even if I had no choices about my physical being.

During his ward rounds, the consultant advised me that the next test would be with the nose and throat department to check whether I had an entry point there for something to enter my brain. Of all the uses I thought of for my nose and throat, entering my brain was not one of them. Again, I managed the procedure by focusing on the moment and relaxing as much as possible with the thought, "I can handle this for five minutes." That is all it took before I returned to the neurology ward. It was yet another situation out of my control but a step forward in the quest to get a diagnosis. In those moments when you lack understanding as to the purpose of tests, try not to feel like a guinea pig.

Most of the time, I was kept in the dark about what the doctors had planned until it was time for the next test, so it was a bit of a surprise when I received word that I would be visiting a scanner unit. I had no idea what the purpose of this test was. The scanner unit was in a part of the hospital that was infrequently visited. It turned out to be the kind of adventure that cemented what came to be my usual phrase, "expect the unexpected." Not in my wildest dreams could I have imagined what was going to happen.

The day of the test arrived. A male nurse built like The Incredible Hulk arrived to take me to the scanner unit. Once I was outside in the waiting area, he disappeared, and I stayed put. A male radiologist wheeled me inside and invited me to sit in a large blue chair. After what seemed like an eternity, he emerged to ask me some personal information and tell me what the test involved.

At that moment, I channelled a prisoner on death row sitting in the electric chair before execution. I managed to reign in my imagination just in time to hear the operative give the final pre-test instructions.

"And then I will give you an injection and call you to go and lie on a couch to do the scan."

Okay, I thought, *got that*. Five minutes later, the radiologist appeared wearing a tabard and carrying what looked like a metal toolbox. I felt as if I had been transported onto the set of a sci-fi movie. The procedure consisted of a radioactive substance injected into my vein. I closed my eyes and fought back the image of the electric chair. After the dose was administered, the man disappeared into the closed room. There was nothing for me to do but wait until I received further instructions. I thought he would come out again, but no, he gave the instructions via a public-address system like being instructed at an airport to proceed to Gate 66.

I tried to get onto the couch with the help of ropes as it was apparent no other human being would come anywhere near me.

The radiologist's voice crackled over the PA system. "Okay, let's begin."

Then the scanner whirred, clicked, and whirred some more.

"Right. Finished. I'll call for someone to collect you."

Another male nurse, not quite as burly as the first, wheeled me back to an isolated area in the ward. Another set of male nurses put me into the bed. I think I got to see every male nurse in the department that day. It didn't dawn on me until later that I had just had a radioactive substance injected and was now considered a health hazard, particularly to female nurses. For the next three days, I was not allowed any visitors, had a separate bathroom, had male nurses only to care for me. At every mealtime, they placed my food on the bedside table at a distance. I would have to bring it closer to eat it, and anything I touched had to be put in individual bags and kept in my space. Curiosity got the best of me, and I took a peek to see what was written on the bags. CAREFUL RADIOACTIVE MATERIAL. I understood immediately and wondered whether that meant I would glow in the dark. Like Lazarus rising from the tomb on the fourth day, I woke up to a familiar routine with familiar female nurses.

The scan allowed the radiologist to observe the areas in my body where the radioactive fluid would be attracted to as those would be areas demanding the most energy. They found three high demand areas: my groin, chest, and head. The medical team debated for a week as to what was next. The respiratory team determined that the risk was too considerable to explore the area in my chest. Surgery in my head was out of the question, so they opted for surgery on the area in my groin as the safest area to investigate. The operation was carried out the following week.

As I was recuperating from the operation, the consultant appeared.

"I'm sorry, but you're still deteriorating."

The rebel in me rose up. "No, I don't agree." I didn't wait for him to react to my boldness. "My body is healing from the surgery, which means the process of healing is still present. If you could give me a little more time in between these tests and surgeries, my body might stand a fighting chance to heal quicker." I surprised myself with my directness, but it was effective. He took my advice.

A few weeks later, after the test results were considered and debated, they planned another invasive test. The aim was to investigate at which stage the red blood cells deteriorated in my body. I was not sure how you could establish that, but I was certain the experts knew of a way to find out. As it turned out, a bone marrow sample would provide the data of where the malfunction originated in the body, whether during or after the creation of red blood cells.

The head nurse held my hand, gently stroking it until the specialist from haematology appeared with her kit. The small stainless-steel trolleys reminded me of the many lumbar punctures I had done. She laid her implements on the table one by one and explained what she would do.

The plan of action was to insert a needle in my bone via my hip and take a sample. Just looking at the size of the needle made my eyes water. The drawn curtains should have given me a clue of what I was in for. The procedure was akin to being kicked by a horse. I had given birth to four children, but my pain level reached its peak during that experience.

I did my best to meditate and focus inward. At the same time, I was keenly aware that my ward mates were getting ready for fish and chips. There I was in the process of an excruciating invasive procedure lamenting the fact that I would miss one of my favourites on the menu.

I was jolted out of my "poor me" feeling by the sound of alarms going off. Suddenly, the ward was sealed off, and a rather bizarre picture emerged. A fellow patient had gone into cardiac arrest. Someone consulted the head nurse, who still happened to be holding my hand as the procedure was ongoing. She explained in no uncertain terms that she could not leave me. The curtains were still drawn, but I figured out the crash team had arrived by all the background noise.

My focus shifted from being concerned about what was going on with me to praying the affected patient would be okay.

"All finished."

The sound of the registrar's voice snapped me

back to attention just in time to see her disappear with her trolley. I got tucked in, brought a sandwich, and then slept all afternoon. Another test completed. The other patient left the ward for care in the cardiac department. She returned a different person weeks later.

Systems are what makes the world go round for me. The more time I spent in the hospital trying to comprehend its system, the more I realized the complexity of how a hospital works as well as how we simply take things for granted until we need to use them. That evening I added a new item to my self-care list: gratitude. I committed to being grateful and expressing gratitude for all the things we take for granted every day during our lifetime.

Thankfulness is a social norm applicable in general situations, while gratitude is the particular manifestation of spirituality, love, and affection. Being grateful is the feeling I had about not having suffered a cardiac arrest, unlike my fellow patient. Being grateful is a feeling while being thankful is an act. When someone does something useful to you, you feel grateful, and you offer your thanks as an action.

I realized then why we gave thanks in church and the meaning behind that gesture. My prayers that night intensified as I expressed gratitude for my life and for the care I received from the doctors and the nurses. I decided each evening before going to sleep, I would thank God too for all the blessings I had received that day.

According to Brother David Steindl-Rast, a Benedictine monk, author, and lecturer, a blessing has two functions: it shows our gratitude for the blessing received as well as honouring the person who gives the grace. It is a connection of giving and receiving, being grateful for the gift, and thankful to the one who gave you that gift.

My gratitude increased, and so did the tests. They seemed never to stop. Like the radioactive scan and exploratory surgeries, they were not all run-of-the-mill tests. The medical team must have been ticking off a list, starting with the most dangerous tests to the benign. They logically worked their way through my body systems and decided I needed a brain biopsy. That meant a return to the teaching hospital by ambulance. A day after arriving, one of the medical students had a brainwave to measure the pressure inside my brain.

I woke up from the procedure to a paparazzi of nurses surrounding my bed, snapping away on their cellphones. *What now*? I wondered. *I must look a right state*, as if appearance was the most important concern at the time. I couldn't figure out why on earth they were taking my picture. Even worse, they seemed oblivious to how I felt about it. I plucked up the courage to ask.

"What are you taking a photo of?"

"Oh, we're just looking at the fox out on the lawn."

Well, that was a reasonable enough explanation. An urban fox gracing the lawn was not an everyday occurrence. *Thank goodness.* Here I thought they were taking pictures of me.

When I looked in the mirror later, I realized the brain biopsy had made me look like I had just had a facelift. My skin was taut, and there were visible staple lines along my hairline. And then I raised my eyes upward. The probe that they inserted into my skull to measure the pressure on my brain looked like a giant jam thermometer. If the competition for attention was between the fox on the lawn and that gigantic thermometer poking out of my head, my money would have been on the thermometer. It was still monitoring the pressure on my brain. Still, neither it nor the biopsy provided an answer to what was going on with my body. The Prof. did not give up, so neither would I.

What the test did do was exclude yet another suspected condition. There was nothing more they could do at the teaching hospital. Back to the medical hospital I went. I admired the tenacity of the doctors in trying to find the cause. Why was I deteriorating, and why was my life ebbing away? Why was the body I thought I knew dissolving? The more invasive the tests became, the longer it took for me to recover from the impact.

The hospital ward was beginning to feel like a second home. It was back to the same old routine of collecting medical data, self-care, and rest. "Keep breathing," I told myself. After all, that's a visible sign that something is still working. My physical body became more challenged, and a conversation took place about the next step: a neck biopsy. It would involve a prior discussion with the neurosurgeon and lots of preparation. I needed time to process and evaluate that conversation. It was a big step.

Discussing it with my husband, he suggested I ask to come home on day release. I did not feel I would be able to take that step and have the procedure done without reminding myself who I was and what I enjoyed the most. We also had an invitation to a 50th birthday garden party, and my husband thought it would be nice to go and do something outside hospital boundaries.

The arrangements for day release were complicated, but I did get permission to go to the party. As I sat in my wheelchair, a man holding a wine glass made his way across the lawn towards me.

"Hi. What happened to put you in a wheelchair?"

His directness put me a little off guard, not in a bad way. Not wanting to give an elaborate answer, I quipped in response.

"All I can say is never be too exciting to consultants in hospitals."

His lips curled into a mischievous grin, and the light went on.

"And you are one, right?" The answer was definite. He went on to explain that he was a neurosurgeon specializing in epilepsy, to which I thought, *that's not what I have*. We continued small talk, and I found him to be a lovely human. I was glad he helped people, other people, and enjoyed my remaining time at the party.

It was a welcome change to participate in a typical normal experience, however painful it was for me physically. It served as a great morale booster. I never mentioned the encounter to my husband. We still had a decision to make about the neck biopsy. I explained my hesitations about this dangerous yet necessary surgery. We agreed to talk again after we had more information, then we could make a decision with all the facts.

5

FLIP THE SWITCH

You can never cross the ocean until you have
the courage to lose sight of the shore.
— André Gide

How could I possibly decide between finding out
what ailed me and losing my life during that
quest? How does a person process that dilemma? I
lay there restless, mostly in tears, not feeling good.
I'll never understand why we need to make crucial
decisions about life or death in such a clinical way.
To the Prof., it might seem the next logical step to
have a neck biopsy done. I, on the other hand, had
seen too many autopsies in detective television
adaptations. I was at this moment feeling like a

sacrificial lamb in the name of science. The decision was so weighty and required prayer.

I feared for my children growing up without their mother. I feared for my husband becoming a widower. The mood got darker and darker, and I cried out in fear to God.

"Why me?" The answer that came back was even more shocking.

"Why not? You are strong, you are faithful, and you need just to relax and trust."

Was that God's voice in my head, or was I hallucinating? Did it even matter? It is the most difficult when you face what could be your last chance at life. Everything becomes crystal clear, and you get to know exactly who you are. If you can see beyond fear, you will see a different picture of yourself emerge.

After days of agonizing, I truly felt that what was happening was awful, but that I would be okay, dead or alive. I still wanted time to prepare and make last-minute arrangements so that my affairs would be in order. I wanted to see my children; I wanted to be amid my family and not decide my fate in a hospital bed. They had put me back in a side room. It disconcerted me a little because one possible explanation was that I was really dying and that the side room provided a peaceful place for family to say their goodbyes. I could choose to die, and the pain of living would be released. I chose life, although that meant the probability of a steep road ahead.

On reflection, it was apparent now that I wanted to live. I decided that whatever happened, I would have to put my trust in God and let go of fixed ideas about how my life was going to unfold. God's timing is different from our timetable, and His perspective includes our entire time on earth. We simply do not have the same angle. As a mother, I would know the outcome of something my children had done wrong before discussing the issue with them. When asking the question of what happened, I usually already knew. It is a similar perspective for our heavenly Father. He knows what has happened and what crossroads we will face in our lives. He knows our purpose, the plan of our life, even if at that moment we have no clue. Trust in the process. The caterpillar must dissolve in the cocoon and have complete trust to transform into the butterfly it will become. As humans, we put our trust in the process that everything will turn out the way it is meant to be. All that is required is trust, gratitude, and faith, even as small as a mustard seed.

The arrangements were made, including a visit

by a solicitor. The meeting settled me. I debated
not telling the children the horror I felt, the pain
of the possibility of leaving them. *Face it*, my inner
voice told me. Only by facing the truth and having
all the facts provided clarity of mind and purpose.

As parents, we had always encouraged the
children to speak and share their fears with us, but
I was not being truthful. Why? I was scared to
death, but I had to find a way to tell them that. I
wanted them to remember me for the mother I
was, a momma bear who is invincible and always
knows what to do. The problem was, that is not
how I felt. I was powerless, scared of dying, and
even more scared to tell them that. I was only 52,
but I believed my time was getting nearer because
I felt so weak. I realized then that the next moment
is never guaranteed. I wanted reassurance, and all
I got were more questions and more disturbing
moments.

Before the children left, I spent a few minutes
telling them each I loved them. I had always had
their back and reassured them everything would
be okay. I wanted to hear the same. I knew they
loved me. That was certain. I told them the
outcome was out of my hands. I had to go through
that ring of fire, and I may not return. In my head,
I pictured the death scene of Denethor from the

movie *The Lord of the Rings*. Denethor, grief-stricken by what he sees as the imminent loss of his son, commands his servants to prepare a funeral pyre for himself and Faramir in Rath Dinén. Denethor stands in the middle of the pyre with a flaming torch in his hand, ready to end it all. Just before he drops the torch to set the pyre ablaze, he declares the ultimate words of defeat, "There is no victory!"

It felt like judgment day. I was so fearful, so incapable of showing them I was afraid, yet deep down in my soul, I knew it was the only way. At that moment, I sought the embrace of the unconditional love of God. Queue dramatic music and a movie scene of a crying woman in a bed clutching at life. There was so much I wanted to share with the ones I loved, so much I wanted to say and do. So much love to give them, so many cuddles to experience. Yet I was staring into the abyss, still feeling the victory would be for the medical profession but not for me. I still felt fear.

Despite the fear, I chose the courage to live. That is the point where you feel you do not know what lies ahead. But I believe you still have a choice. You need to hang onto the will to live if that is your choice. I was begging for my life, and it was not pretty. I was trying to make a pact that if I lived, I would start again. Like a naughty child, I reevaluated whatever wrong I thought I'd done and promised never to do it again. I kept listening for the Shepherd's staff tapping on the rocks.

> Even though I walk through the darkest valley, I will fear no evil, for you are with me; your rod and staff, they comfort me.
> — Psalm 23 v4 NIV

I would follow, I would find peace, I would sleep and rest. I pictured Jesus on the cross, and at that moment, I understood. In some respects, it felt the same, although I had a different cross to bear. I was nailed to the medical cross. I had to find the courage to submit to God's will and not mine. I had made the choice to live, but I was still floating in and out of consciousness without much awareness. *Was I dying?* We all get nailed to a cross in moments like those when we face the fear of dying.

After a while, I woke up. My time was up. A transfer to the teaching hospital was imminent, and I had to make a decision. I felt helpless, but strangely at peace. My dark night of the soul had passed. I just had to relax. My husband took my hand and did his best to reassure me.

"It will be alright in the end. And if not, then it's not the end."

That's when I saw he was scared too. He was trying to put on a brave face.

"We are in this together," he said.

I felt the love and a definite feeling of floating in an embrace of love. *Dying is not that bad*, I thought, and then drifted off into nowhere again.

In between moments of conscious, a message from a card I received from my friend popped into my mind:

> If you cannot see the light at the end of the tunnel, for goodness sake, walk down there and flip the switch.

I had to be determined to find the switch. Nothing is impossible. The word itself spells out I AM POSSIBLE (with a little creative license, of course). I had to find that switch if it was the last thing I did. I recalled the words that all is possible with God. You spend a lifetime listening to the terms, but they never quite become meaningful until they do.

All the while, I had more care and attention from the nurses. Their movements were mechanical and urgent. They smiled, but there were no lines around their eyes. Their words were cheerful, but a minor note was undeniable. The monitors beeped, and my bedside was flanked by medical staff. The world blanked out, and I became unconscious again. When I came to, I agreed to talk to the neurosurgeon, making it clear it would be a fact-finding mission. It took days to be stable enough to travel, but the day finally arrived.

My daughter met me at the appointment. As we entered his consulting room, I felt great relief to be accompanied by a trusted family member who could listen to the conversation. From the patient's perspective, we hear only a fraction of the discussion. We are just not fully capable of processing the words fast enough to comprehend. We are a ball of nerves, have flashes of fear, and are usually not in the best mental or emotional place to make vital decisions. It is essential to have a person you trust and who knows how you think to act as a sounding board to revisit what was said at the consultation.

As we looked at the imaging of the inside of my body, the neurosurgeon explained what he wanted to do. The risks involved were immense.

"To be honest, it means going far deeper in your neck than I am comfortable to do."

Those were the words that stuck. I returned to my hospital bed in tears. The surgery could be successful and provide an answer, or I could survive in a vegetative state needing round the clock care and barely functioning. Or I could die on the operating table. What choices to have. I prayed about it over the next few days and decided that whatever happened, I would be okay. I recalled, "the Lord is my Shepherd." Even when we cannot sense His presence, we can hear the knocking of the staff against the rocks. Following the sound, the sheep will get safely through the pass. I had to trust and not imagine adverse outcomes. I accepted the neurosurgeon was skilled and would do the best he could, but I could not commit to having the procedure done at that time.

More tests followed. Three months later, I had another appointment with Prof. He asked if there was any change as to whether I would consider the neurosurgery again. I confirmed it had. Still, I wanted time to put my affairs in order, discuss this with my children, and protect my family. All this while I was feeling like rubbish and crying a lot. The worst-case scenario for me would not be death, but to end up in a vegetative state. I wanted to give my husband the authority to make decisions about my care legally. It was so intense, so personal, so painful, and so final.

To support myself as best I could, I continued with all my self-care daily and spent a great deal of time in meditation and conversation with God. I asked the medical team for time to get my act together, and after six weeks, I was ready. I was scared and grateful for the life I had, but I couldn't help wondering if I was expecting the worst yet hoping for the best.

I took the time to tell my family how much I loved them and how much they meant to me. It was reminiscent of a soldier going to fight in battle. I was unsure whether I would see them again in this lifetime. Then, like a grenade tossed into the camp before you have a chance to pick up your rifle, an emergency followed, which transferred me straight to the teaching hospital before the scheduled date. Time was up. The ultimate decision was made and out of my hands. I had no other option but to put my trust in God. I kept breathing, kept calm, and felt horrible, but I now know God was with me. I floated in and out of awareness, barely cognizant of what would happen next.

We always discuss matters that create a challenge as a family because we all have different perspectives and solutions. The reason our children talk to us is that we communicate with them even if the subject is complicated or difficult. As humans, we generally shy away from frank discussions about challenging issues. Yet, no progress can be made until we honestly and openly discuss perspectives within a trusted relationship, whether that be family, a counselor, a medical professional, or a chaplain. It is our best option to find a solution that can bring us peace. Give yourself time to talk it over with a person who not only shows you unconditional love, but who also knows you as a person and with whom you feel safe and respected.

6

GOD IS IN THE DETAILS

Seek goodness everywhere, and when it is found, bring it out of its hiding place and let it be free and unashamed.
— William Saroyan

"I did not think she would make it," the ambulance driver later admitted. In hindsight, I imagine I must have looked a fright. They kept me on hold in a quiet ward in the teaching hospital where Prof. was visiting me. I cannot believe how cheeky I could be. Facing death has a way of divorcing you from other people's opinions. I said what I wanted because I had nothing to lose.

Prof. told me he was 90 percent certain he had

nailed down what the problem was. Still, he did not want me to receive medication until he was sure.

"Why don't you try medication?" I said. "If it works, you will be right, and if not, it's the other option."

He did not respond to that, which provoked exasperation.

"If you don't find out soon, the pathologist will find the answer post-mortem and get all the credit!"

Well, that did not get the response I'd hoped for. Prof. confirmed that I would have to have a neck biopsy. Ouch! I was still scared to death of that. Then it slowly dawned on me that I could be so near the end anyway, it would not matter. I would have to go ahead.

"Okay, you win."

Within hours the neurosurgeon arrived at my bedside. *Hold on. It's a different man.* Yet I was sure I had heard this concerned voice before.

He took my hand and promised to look after me. I talked about my concerns, and he reassured me he would be back later that day. A few hours later, the masked man was no longer in scrubs. He held what looked to me like astronomy charts.

"Don't worry if you wake up in an iron lung, because where I need to be is millimetres from the nervous system that controls your breathing."

Was this what he called reassuring me? I was terrified at that thought. I calmed down a little by reminding myself that I would be under anaesthesia and wouldn't know anything about what was happening anyway. At least, not until I woke up. He took my hand again, promising to take away everything that did not belong in the neck space.

"I have cleared my schedule, and the surgery will take place first thing tomorrow."

And then it dawned on me as if my subconscious mind had finally completed its voice recognition and matched it to a face in my memory. It was the man I'd met on the garden lawn with a wine glass in his hand. He had the same knowing look on his face. It was a chance meeting that would become a vital one. That moment was when being scared turned into a sacred moment, just as quickly as you could change the letters around.

My perception of time was not God's perception of time. My path had crossed with the chosen surgeon who would carry out this critical procedure. At that realization, I thanked God for taking my fear away and delivering me into the hands of a surgeon who was handpicked to perform this procedure. I fell asleep with a sense of peace and thankfulness. It was out of my hands, and the prospect gave me peace rather than terror. *Trust the process*. That was my last thought before falling asleep.

The next morning at six, preparations began for surgery. I offered a prayer of thanks to God, a God I had never entirely accepted as being a real consideration in my life before all this happened. That moment, a relationship with God that had been missing clicked into place. As the anaesthesia took its effect, I slowly fell asleep, knowing my life was in His hands, and the surgeon would do the best he could. I had tried everything up until that moment, and I needed to surrender. It's interesting to me now that even though I had only gone through the motions at church, the last words to register in my mind were, "Anything is possible with God."

When I woke up, the nurses told me the surgery lasted nine hours. I wondered how it went. I did not see an iron lung, so I believed that it had gone as well as could be expected. The nurses transferred me to the intensive care unit where two nurses provided individual around the clock care. I was as quiet as a mouse but praying silently and giving thanks.

7

THE SHUT GATE

The beginning is always today.
— Mary Wollstonecraft Shelley

"I made a mistake," said the anaesthetist.

I was lying in bed, peacefully minding my own business, when the young man in scrubs appeared. He approached my bedside in a manner I can only describe as a combination of fear and embarrassment.

His voice was trembling. "I have come to apologize because I made a mistake during the surgery."

He had my attention. "Hmm."

I'm not a vindictive person, and whenever my

children would say they were sorry, I would ask what had happened to cause their mistake.

"What happened?"

He shuffled from one foot to the other and took a visual scan from the ceiling to the floor before he landed his eyes back on me. "Yes. Well, because the surgery took longer than expected, I may have caused damage to your left eye."

"What? You managed to destroy a part of my body that was not already damaged. How could you do such a thing?"

"I am so sorry. I should have taped your eyes shut so as to not dry them out during surgery."

The damage was done. The patient disappeared, and the mother in me surfaced as I asked him what he had learned from the experience. He assured me it would stay with him during his career, and he would not make that mistake again.

"That's good enough for me. Just make sure it does not happen again." And then, as if talking to the anaesthetist had the same effect as his administration, I fell promptly asleep again, drained from all the emotion.

I still did not receive medication because the tissues taken from the biopsy would need further investigation. Frankly, I had no idea how long that would take, but it was no longer as important. I felt in safe hands, in a way that passed my understanding. I was in a lot of pain yet also relieved of all the emotional pain and anxiety. I felt like a child that is aware of the unconditional love of a parent.

Although I had been aware of God's presence in my life, it was as if I had been standing in a dry pasture looking at God standing in a lovely meadow. Why on earth I could not be over there with Him was beyond my comprehension. Little did I understand I would have to open the gate. I had always seen the gate as locked, and all it took was for me to go and open that gate and walk into the meadow of my own free will. The realization it was unlocked and also open began my awareness that we often take a restriction as imposed by others. There was never a restriction in place. What if all it takes is to go and try to open the gate? What if all it takes is for us to use our free will?

My life would never be the same again, but the fact I was here, recovering in the intensive care ward, meant it would be alright. "Hold on." That's what my husband had said. It would not be the end.

8

ENDLESS PATIENCE

Face reality as it is, not as it was or as you wish it
to be.
— Jack Welch

Life in a hospital has its rhythms. When we are too
poorly to notice, we submit to how things are. Life
for the patient is, for the most part, out of our
control. Yet, the routine of the hospital
environment provides structure and a steady
rhythm that contains our chaotic world.

The sun shines through the window, casting
sun shadows over the bedclothes. You get used to
regular checks, blood tests, hospital routines, and
nurses visiting you daily. You wonder when, even
if, you are ever going to leave the hospital. You

have an extra regular visitor in the cleaner who comes on schedule and cleans your room and the small bay you occupy.

Having a single room might be an advantage for peace. However, being on a shared ward opens the opportunity to observe and entertain. There will be more people to see as well as having absolute solidarity with your fellow patients, whereas being in a single room might seem lonely.

In certain circumstances, whether you are in a ward or not very much depends on your medical needs. Each environment, shared or solitary, offers different perspectives and opportunities for growth. Being in a single room provides privacy when you have visitors. As I enjoy all music, it brought a feeling of being in my space where I was able to play my music, even at 3 a.m., when sleep evaded me. I could sleep when the rest of the world would be buzzing with activity.

There will be a moment with a spinal injury where you are not yet recovered nor in need of medical attention. You may be tempted to entertain the thought that you might never leave this space. Allow your thoughts to swing toward the positive side of the "what if" pendulum. Remain focused on the professional disciplines at work to prepare you for living, leaving, and moving into a safe place where your care continues.

Despite being bed-bound and unable to move independently, the physiotherapist would visit regularly and move my legs. Other days the occupational therapist encouraged movement through little tasks that strengthened different muscles. I became quite adept at big wooden puzzles and exercising and breathing on a smaller scale. I could only go for short periods as I had very little energy. With repetitive movements, however small, the response of your muscles gets stronger over time.

Over the months, my care needs changed. I was slowly reclaiming the ability to direct my attention to small tasks I could undertake, first under supervision, and when safe, alone. The first time I could lift my sippy cup to my mouth was like winning Olympic gold. I learned to celebrate the small victories while keeping a vision in my awareness as to where I wanted to be. Having studied as an early educator specializing in children from the age of 0-7, I knew what milestones I had to achieve linearly to progress. We learn different skills at each developmental level. A child follows an internal program pointing towards the next developmental stage. I had to do the same and link into that process.

After the neck surgery, my body behaved like a newborn. I had no control over the movement of my head. It was so heavy and needed support. I had no muscle strength. When I tried to lift my head from my shoulders, it would not budge, just lolled about. The surgery had damaged my spinal cord, and at that point, I didn't know if the damage was temporary or permanent.

Gradually, I progressed to holding my fork and guiding food towards my mouth. Walking was simply many stages ahead and would require carefully inbuilt exercises and activities to reach those little milestones. As I reached each developmental milestone, the therapists would introduce new equipment and exercises: ball games, puzzles, smaller and smaller objects more substantial in weight, etc. It seemed never-ending. Your physical ability will get you to a certain level where the therapists will discuss moving you to a different setting. With more advanced abilities, you will transfer to another supportive rehab setting to continue your recovery.

I have always encouraged my children to follow their dreams, no matter how out of reach they may seem. I would encourage them to reflect on what they could do today to take the next step towards that vision. First, as a useful activity, you may wish to practice creating a vision board with everything you would ideally want in your new life. Not everything will be immediately possible, but over time, with baby steps, you will find the inner guidance to get as close as possible to it.

My vision board was a stick and paste exercise done with the help of the occupational therapist. I would point to the pictures in the magazines, she would cut them, put glue on them, and I would place them on my image in ever-increasing ability. The final collage had all the favourable colours, everything essential I visualized in my future. I had many personal memorial services as I mourned the loss of my life as I once knew it and embraced a level of acceptance of how things would be. Certain things I loved to do would not be able to be achieved. I would return to them and examine precisely what that activity's reward was and how that reward could be received in another way. More details on that later.

After the doctors have diagnosed what needs to be done to make you feel better and start to feel better, the question of when you can go back home and pick up life where you left off may arise. That process involves a lot of work. The hospital staff's priority is to keep you safe and well. They will help you build up your strength and resilience to a point where you can be transferred to a safe location. Ideally, that place is your home, but not necessarily.

The neck biopsy had provided the name of what had caused all this destruction: a rare neurological condition called neurosarcoidosis. My best explanation is that it forms clusters of white blood cells that settle anywhere in the body and cause disruption or permanent damage in random locations in the body. In my case, the neurosarcoidosis damaged or limited most of my functions below the waist, confining me to a wheelchair. This is described as an incomplete spinal injury caused by disease (incomplete as there is some function). It is considered a non-traumatic injury as it was not caused by a sudden event but progressed slowly. Medical professionals call it non-traumatic. But I would question how a spinal injury could ever be considered "non-traumatic."

Although my condition was now known and I received some treatment for it, I was certainly not well enough to leave. How long was never mentioned, and life in a rehabilitation ward became my reality.

Over the months, I would gradually work on a prescribed exercise program and have conversations about my home and the care I would need. The conversations can seem a bit overwhelming, and it is perfectly okay to feel everything from anger, frustration, sadness, etc. Every day I would do my little self-care routine, listen to music, and pour my emotions out to God and into my journal.

The beauty of the journal is that even when you think you are not progressing, you are. On the other hand, God is a good and faithful listener. Thoughts are great as a process, but pouring those thoughts on paper in a journal provides extra depth and dimension. Doodling, colouring, drawing, cutting, sticking and pasting, and writing are different expressions that originate in our inner being. You can check what life was like a few months ago. Whenever you feel you are not doing anything and getting nowhere, the journal will surprise you and offer hope in the strangest of ways.

To know that three months prior, I could not hold the weight of my neck and now could turn my head gives that little glimmer of hope that things heal and change. Time heals, and change happens gradually, though progress may not be linear. For every three steps I took in a forward direction, I would invariably have a setback. Three steps forward and two back still become one step ahead, albeit very, very slowly.

Slow and steady are good, and feedback is just feedback. It does not mean to say that things will not change. It means you must try to approach things more gradually and have more patience.

The physiotherapist continued to exercise my limbs. My rolling in the bed improved, and the strength in my arms increased enough for me to use a Rota stand and sit in the chair for fifteen minutes a day to have lunch. My power increased slowly, and standing on a Rota stand was manipulated by two nurses. Although very unimportant compared to walking, it became an outstanding achievement compared to sleeping in a bed for twenty hours a day. At least the time passed quickly. The way you evaluate progress depends on what your comparison is. My son told me to forget the future and concentrate on the next baby step. Hard to do if you are a goal-oriented personality, but little by little, I got the hang of it.

I received more intravenous medication. I made slow progress in reversing the neurosarcoidosis that attacked my body and had paralyzed me from the waist down. It had damaged my spine and had inflamed my brain stem, making many functions erratic, broken, or seemingly impossible. The body, however, did so well at keeping it all together. I had accused it many times of letting me down. Yet, it had valiantly supported me throughout the whole period. It was a process of transformation.

Eventually, we got to the point where there was no progression of the illness. The damage to my body stabilized. At that moment, I looked like a complete car wreck, but at least no one was continually trying to crash my engine or hit my head against a brick wall. I told myself, "If I have survived this far, surely I am going to survive, and it will get better."

During the next few months, the pace of recovery intensified. I transferred to a recovery hospital whose sole task seemed to be to prepare me for reentering into the world outside the hospital's sterile walls.

I had various notebooks creating a process of questions that would enable me to live my best life under the circumstances. Getting to an acceptable level where leaving the hospital seems a possibility is a very long, carefully thought out process. The physiotherapist and occupational therapist do not want you to go home and struggle without someone there to support you. They know where you want to be and how long you must be in the hospital before leaving them.

The team continually plan and assess where you are. You think you might be ready and chomping at the bit, yet you may not have all the facts. Your home environment may need adaptations; you may need equipment to manage; you and your family need to be ready. The circumstances that make it possible for you to have a lousy day must be in place at home so that care and recovery can continue. The more complex your needs are, the more challenging and work-intensive their planning needs to be. Time is immaterial. You may well feel that you are ready, but their perspective may be different.

The team finally had the conversation which introduced the concept of me going back home. It was impossible physically to move in. The building was ancient, with winding staircases and floors at different levels. The things I loved most about my home made it impossible for me to live there as the new me. That was a harsh realization as our homes are a reflection of and part of our personality. When our needs change, it follows that our home environment might have to change too.

The decision by the support team was that I would have to go into a residential facility. I said no, that was not my vision. I was in my early 50s. I had three children at home and a husband, altogether a caring family unit. I had not just gone through this ordeal to then live a separated life. I preferred a future in which I made my own choices as against living in an institution.

It is necessary to accept that the health support team will do its best to make sure you receive adequate care and comfort. At the same time, you have opportunities to make your voice heard too. You have preferences and a vision of your future by now. That vision is realistic, wanting to enjoy life as much as possible within the boundaries set. I missed my friends too. My family and a few friends mainly supported me. I started to notice I enjoyed their company and their interest in making me feel positive and better. Despite everything, I kept my sense of humour, and we had good times in a hospital ward, laughing and joking. My friendships transformed from many superficial ones to a few deep mutual ones. They say when something terrible happens, you will find out who your friends are.

Happiness is a state we achieve when our expectations meet our reality. If I had insisted on seeing the future as my pre-illness self, deep unhappiness would have been a daily occurrence. I was termed as disabled, yet I saw the opportunity to be differently able. True, there are things I cannot do, but with adaptation, I can do them differently. Every day in recovery is a chance to weigh what you need to do and how you are supported to achieve that. Your journal will provide information about the progress you are making. It's time to be authentic as well as realistic. You will eventually emerge as the butterfly you are. The journal is a tool to harness in words what you want your reality to be.

People often use the phrase "Rome was not built in a day." When you become differently able, it becomes even more apparent that important work takes time. You can investigate how you can do all the essential things differently. Anything else that is not critical for the moment can be done in the future. What you cannot do today, you may do differently tomorrow.

9

BICYCLES AND BRUISES

And suddenly you know; it's time to start
something new and trust the magic of new
beginnings.
— Meister Eckhart

After months of building up muscles to tackle the
Rota stand, walking seemed an impossible task,
yet I was determined to do so. Every few days, I
would be taken to the parallel bars and made to
stand up hanging from a harness supporting my
body. All I could see in my mind was the harness I
used to strap my babies in that would hang from
the door. It would strengthen their muscles as well
as condition their bodies to be upright. My
turn now.

I stood at the bars for maybe a few minutes and tried so much to stand up. What was to be a joyous moment of standing upright was laced with the realization I had no feeling, no response, no connection from the waist down. There was a deep sadness to overcome as well as gratefulness. At least the legs were still there. Even without functional legs, I was grateful to have the love and strength to carry on life with all it has to offer.

Fast forward a few weeks where I spent time in meditation towards acceptance that walking would be just about impossible. During this, a man arrived with a tape measure to measure my hips. *Another undignified moment* I thought, having never really loved my body because it was pear-shaped and at its fullest at the bones. And I let that go, fascinated by the fact they measured my hips.

Over the next few weeks, I would visualize the concept of the wheelchair.

"You can handle the wheelchair," said the occupational therapist with a smile. The remark was intended to sound like good news, but to my ears, it had the ring of a life sentence.

The wheelchair arrived as a gift that would improve my mobility. It would move me from my room and offer possibilities to get around. It was a standard wheelchair as it only provided the opportunity to be taken somewhere else by someone pushing me in it. I hated the concept, and I never wanted to be in a wheelchair, let alone be driven by someone else. I was an independent woman, a mother of four children. Why on earth would I be delighted to be in a wheelchair?

During a rare visit from my youngest son, he commented that maybe I was looking at this scenario the wrong way. I felt anger telling myself, how would he know? He's just a 12-year-old, fully able kid with all his hopes and dreams intact. But he got my attention.

"What do you mean?"

"Well, Mum, it's not a wheelchair, you see. It's a bike. It will get you from A to B, and that's what a bicycle does."

What a refreshing point of view that immediately changed the perspective. Seeing it as a wheelchair was terrible news because of all my negative images and feelings associated with it. When the mental image turned into a bike, suddenly, the sense of freedom I had felt cycling around my neighbourhood and in nature transformed the experience.

"Yes, that's so much better. Thank you. I will look at it as a bike."

The wheelchair was ceremoniously presented

one day with the directive I would have to build up to sitting in it at various times of the day. Yes, it was a bike, but a very ugly one with neck support built on.

The tipping point to go home was to be able to spend time on that bike and get through the day. In the months following, the aim was to spend up to eight hours in it, be taken around the hospital, participate in activity sessions, and, more importantly, exercise sessions. They were trying to broaden my sphere. It was immensely tiring to sit up, and there were only so many times I had the energy to transfer to bed from the wheelchair. The best practical advice and techniques I found were by watching Richard Corbett from *Wheels2Walking* and Gem Hubbard from *Wheelsnoheels*.

One of the big family treats was that it enabled me to leave the hospital on special leave to join the family and enjoy a pizza meal. It had been planned carefully for weeks. There was a hiccup, however. My wheelchair was too large to get in the wheelchair taxi. With the determination of the younger me squeezing myself into a much smaller pair of jeans, I pretended to be comfortable. After all, I did not physically feel a thing. And meeting the boys and their dad was too important to me. So, I had a mediocre evening where indeed, I could not eat as it squeezed my insides to the max. How I would get out of the chair was beyond me, but they would work it out. Spending time eating pizza sitting around the table was my first go at normality. It was anything but ordinary, but I had been looking forward to the evening so much. I came back by taxi, thrilled and utterly exhausted.

They did eventually pry the wheelchair from my body. It was well and truly stuck. As I stood on the Rota stand, the wheelchair would rise with me. The next morning would reveal bruises on either side of my upper legs. There was no mention of it the following day, and I understood that the evening madness would not happen again. Nonetheless, I had spent an evening with my family, and that was a remarkably high reward for me. I slept for days.

Finding the perfect matched wheelchair for your needs takes a little time. You must be comfortable. It must fit your size, your home, and your lifestyle. The first chair was to enable someone else to push me around. Gradually I wanted to build up muscle strength to self-propel the wheelchair. I practiced little steps of improvement each day. I was increasing weight training by using tins or water bottles filled with an incremental volume of water. It was plodding progress, but I was not disheartened. If you keep a vision in your mind and take little steps toward it each day regularly, keeping notes in your journal, you will see incremental progress. No matter how small, it's progress.

After months, my husband managed to find a suitable property for us to move to that included a bathroom more suitable for someone with a disability. I would never be able to go upstairs, and the dining room downstairs was equipped with a hospital bed. The opportunity to go home in my environment with my wheelchair became possible. I was overjoyed! Even if I would mostly have to stay home, I would be able to interact with my family.

The occupational therapist visited the home and planned for all equipment needed for my care and comfort to be in situ. When everything was in place, they had to test my response to everything at home. Care visits happened four times a day, a daily routine organized, and with their confidence satisfied, they took me to the new house.

After two years in hospital, returning to a new home took energy I did not have. Initially, I struggled to stay well despite visits by caregivers daily. Do not underestimate how dependent you become on the hospital routine and the continuity of caring staff. At home, I saw up to fifteen caregivers per week, my food changed, and I was a bit lost as to what I would be doing all day. I found that the little routine I had developed in the hospital served me well. I took an interest in the caregivers visiting me. Every day I would look at something that frustrated me and patiently work a way for it to be better. Making the most of it, I think they call it. "This or better" became my guiding motto. Working diligently with the journal did provide answers within my being in time. Not always immediately, but visiting it every day provided a routine as well as a safe space to process my thoughts, ideas, fears, and other feelings.

You will probably get a whole list of equipment delivered to your home, and they will make suggestions for adaptations if needed. It can be overwhelming. I did not want my house to look like a disabled home either inside or outside. I had children who lived at home, so I chose a part of the home that would mainly be for me. I left them as much of the house untouched so they would be able to call it their home. I did not want them to see it as assisted living accommodation.

It's crucial to know that my disability is different from yours. That means that the equipment and setting out of your home will be unique to you and your circumstances. To be honest, there are times where it's easier to let the therapists get on with their plan, even if you feel frustrated. There will be opportunities to make changes. They aim to get you home with the equipment you need and the care you need to stay stable. You might be keen to get back home, but too many objections and obstructions put up by you even for the best of reasons can cause delays.

Staying out of hospital will gradually allow you to make baby step changes to your environment. You will no doubt feel a little overwhelmed by the changes. In my case, the toll was emotional as well. I was happy to be out of the hospital but a little apprehensive about life ahead.

10

SHIFTING GEARS

One foot, then the other. Don't look at all five
feet at once. Just take a step. And when you've
taken that step, take one more. Eventually, you'll
make it to the shower. And you'll make it to
tomorrow and next year too. One step.
— Lori Gottlieb

As children, we have had an experience of care,
good, indifferent, or wrong. That experience in
your mind will be the understanding with which
you approach the care offered. Plans need to be
put in place to best care for you away from a
hospital environment. If your care needs are high,
there will be options to move into a residential
care facility. On the other end of the scale, you

might move into an environment where you can live independently but with support on hand, or move back home. It's crucial to make your case as to what is important to you and how that can translate into a care option and closest match to all your requirements and budget.

Health professionals must ensure that your home environment is suitable for your return. Mine was not. The first alternative they offered was to go into residential care. Still, as I am very independent, I fought hard against living in an institution. My family was at home, and that was the environment in which I was most comfortable. Then I applied for assisted housing but, although successful, would have had to live on my own without my family, which again was not my preferred option. A few weeks later, my husband described a home in the vicinity, much smaller but accessible. Although bijou, it offered the best solution for us.

It's essential to contemplate how you see your care and environment and advocate for that option. I wanted to be independent. I tried to find a new direction since I was now differently able, but I would need to plan that course in my imagination and the action steps needed to obtain the desired outcome.

I had used vision boards myself as well as with my clients. All future goals and wishes would be put on a board to view daily. I looked at various magazines and, this time around, cut out meaningful pictures and words using children's scissors. It took a few weeks, but I ended up with a clear vision of the next step, how I wanted my future to look. I completed the second vision board by myself with little help. Progress.

A residential facility, although probably more comfortable to transition to from the hospital's point of view, was not my perspective. I did discuss it with them giving my reasons, and they compromised after some debating. My husband knew me best and continuously supported me. He would advocate for me if anything were suggested that would make me unhappy.

It is a long process to find harmony between your needs and your preferences. It is, however, not impossible. If you can, persevere, revisit, do your homework, find out the criteria that need to be matched and make a proposal. It will, no doubt, be adjusted. The hospital staff may advise you that they do not do it that way. Still, you need to find an approach to what suits you, not their vision but an environment that suits your needs. Transferring to a residential facility might be convenient for your safety, but how do you envisage managing your life in the future? Who are you now? What do you want to do? How do you want to live within the limitations and restrictions presented? It is a unique answer that needs careful consideration and planning. It takes time, and you can always reconsider. No decision is final, and they will always respect your wishes, depending on the costs involved.

I chose to go back to my family in a new smaller home. What was most important to us was to be together as a family to support me. It would allow me the opportunity to continue to have an input in my children's lives, which was my reason for living. What is yours? What is most important to you?

The staff prepared everything for me to move into my new home. It was a new beginning as well as a new care routine. The first experience of home care was after I had my stroke years previously. A man showed up at my home. When my husband answered the door, he felt uncomfortable showing another man into our bedroom. He had no idea the caregiver would be male. I needed help having a shower, and all that went through my mind was that at some point, I would have to undress in front of another man. I kept apologizing to the caregiver, saying it was me, not him. I had to change my perspective, and I would. It took time.

The second time around needing care, my plan required four visits daily by two caregivers just for my basic needs, up to fifteen different people per week. Although it provided reassurance and continuity of care, I had to adapt to different caregivers doing things in different ways. Each team was unique in its approach to reaching the objectives set. Again, it took time: male teams, female teams, mixed teams, young as well as more experienced caregivers. Any combination you could imagine.

It sort of worked a little clunky at the beginning. Months passed, and I was in no position to consider alternatives, although there are alternatives to research and consult. I am immune suppressed, and therefore, more vulnerable. Meeting fifteen different people who can visit up to twenty different people in a day increases my exposure to three hundred. For that reason, I opted to be cared for by a small team of regular caregivers and currently have three, seven days a week.

Let me explain the principle of the spoon theory I use to manage my energy. Spoons are a visual representation of energy units. Every day you are given x-number of spoons. Let's say I have fifteen spoons. Getting up and getting dressed would be equivalent to three spoons. Eating my meals, another three spoons. Transferring from the wheelchair, two spoons, watching a film, two spoons, a little garden work, two spoons, a nurse takes blood, one spoon, clothes change, one spoon, making a drink, one spoon, and voila, all my spoons are gone.

The spoon theory allows you to dissect your day into doing three necessary tasks and then add less important activities. If you have any energy units after that, you can use them at your leisure. Some activities are more energy-intensive and require more energy than others. If my day is extremely demanding, I will plan a light menu to enable my digestive system to use less energy than usual and back up the extra demands in energy. Not getting the balance right results in collapse. That, of course, is to be avoided. There are days you can bank a spoon and days you can give up a spoon to recover, but it's a careful balance to consider.

Since my way of working prior to this was similar to a bull in a china shop, moving forward like a mild pussycat took some getting used to.

Every action was a careful management of energy. A visit to the hairdresser involves energy to get in the taxi. Having my hair cut means making allowances to ensure I use no more than my allocated spoons. I could add a spoon by sleeping for one hour, but that would be like replenishing energy with a faulty charger. I had a full schedule before my illness, and I was always moving at rapid speed, so it took me a while to adjust to the principles of the spoon theory.

Spoons are not just units of physical energy, but mental and emotional energy too. That explained why attending a parents' evening at my son's school was so taxing. Physical strength to get there, brain power to pay attention and concentrate, and the emotional energy expended because I was so proud of my son all took their toll.

Until I understood the spoon theory, I often ended up exhausted, wondering what had happened to get me there. I allocate all spoons when I feel well, all things considered. On bad days I only give myself twelve spoons (three less than normal) to enable my body to recover. With the spoon theory's help, I managed to rebuild a fulfilling life, and you will be able to in time.

Even though my body has changed beyond

recognition, the essence of who I am is still there, and I am trying to keep as healthy as possible. All those days in bed, working with my journal, helped me understand. I needed to find a way to continue to express who I was and decided in the first years of adaptation and recovery that I would become differently able.

Being "disabled" concentrated on not being able to do things and, in my opinion, is a negative that gets continuously repeated. Being uniquely capable means that you can focus on doing something even if it's with difficulty compared to how most people do things. You can be creative and find different ways to get the job done. Sometimes it requires ultra-creative thinking, and sometimes you fail at the task, but at least you would have tried. Allow me to inspire you with a few examples.

- If you cannot read because the level of concentration required and holding a book is detrimental to your health management, consider audiobooks.
- If watching a film and going to the cinema was a pleasure that now seems impossible, how about watching it on your computer and getting a loved one

to bring popcorn and watch it
with you.

- If you liked to go places and visit
  museums and new cities, why not visit
  them virtually on a computer from
  your wheelchair.
- Make a cup of tea independently. If you
  cannot lift a regular-sized kettle, get
  one that makes a cup, and use a travel
  mug so you can take the tea with you
  without scalding yourself.

Another example, which is a personal
favourite, is swimming. I love swimming, but that
would require transport to the facility, a caregiver
to undress and dress me, exercise, and
transportation back. I am not able to do that.
However, the feeling of running water on my body
(as in a long refreshing shower) is possible at
home. Add luxury products, sitting in a shower
wheelchair, being dried in fluffy towels, you end
up smelling fabulous, and having a spa
experience. It engages all my senses (those I can
connect with anyway). It's an activity that I can
experience at home, though not every day since
the simple act of taking a shower uses two of my
fifteen spoons. The risk of using the two spoons is

sometimes worth the reward of feeling refreshed, clean, and incredible after the event.

My way of approaching an action from a different angle is to weigh the reward against the risk involved. Then using metaphoric spoons as units of energy, I find a way to do it. And here is the key: just because you can do it does not mean you have to do it. You end up living more mindful, being present in the moment.

Before my injury, I was a multi-tasking woman with four children. I never sat still and accomplished everything I wanted. In the eyes of everyone else, I acted like I was a successful wonder woman. Full-time job, commute, gym, etc. If one of the children required a cake or fancy-dress costume, I would make it even at late notice. Listening to what I did in a week then would exhaust me now.

What was it like after the injury? It felt a bit like wading through molasses. It was frustrating having something as simple as making a cup of tea take an hour, and my body would see that as a monumental task. Things that were a breeze before were so tricky now.

Michael Nobbs, artist, podcaster, and founder of Go Gently, encourages doing just one thing a day. Michael has Myalgic encephalomyelitis (ME), also known as chronic fatigue syndrome (CFS), a chronic illness that severely limits how much he can do each day. He has shown me how to bring simple pleasures into my daily life despite minimal energy. He inspired me to adopt the "one thing a day" principle. If anything, achieving that one thing, reframing your expectations, and celebrating the little achievements, built a sense of accomplishment.

Instead of being faced daily with disappointment at not being able to do anything, the one thing a day schedule brought focus, attention, and achievement. It encouraged me to celebrate the little victories. The activities were broken down into 10-minute chunks of time that were doable and achievable. Michael uses a timer, and when it rings, wherever he is in the activity, he stops and rests. It became a way to acknowledge that tasks broken down in small chunks of time could be done and no longer felt impossible.

Not until I grasped the principle of one thing a day did my body relax enough to think, okay, I can do that. Before, I used to take a quick shower before work every day, but now I faced the prospect of being washed in bed, yet I wanted to have a shower. I received the help of an occupational therapist who told me it might take months to get to have a shower, but we would work on it. "Okay," I replied. "Let's do this." The first task was to sit up in bed, and we practiced that for a week. Then I had to figure out, with her help, how I would swing my legs out of the bed.

The nano steps towards anything were a mammoth task. Each undertaking would leave me exhausted, but over the weeks, my confidence to do these tasks increased. I was not allowed to go to the next step until I had mastered the previous one without too much effort. We practiced swinging the legs to get out of bed for three months using various techniques. The ultimate achievement was to then transfer to a shower chair, which was not too different from practicing transfers into the wheelchair. Finally, I could have a shower, and after eight months, I was over-excited. After having it, I was utterly exhausted.

My plan to have my daily shower, such a big part of my morning routine before the injury, suddenly consumed most of my energy and left me unable to function. To have a shower every day was just not possible. We had to start with one shower a month, then two, then three. Eventually, one shower a week. Each shower was like having a little victory and needed a celebration. I currently manage two showers a week, use luxury shower products, and soft fluffy towels in my preferred colour. It ends up being a spa experience, followed by resting for the majority of the day.

One day my son saw that I was still getting frustrated by the many tasks I had to learn to do.

"Mum, trust the process. Don't look at the top of the staircase as to how far you still need to get. Concentrate on the next step and only on the step in front of you. Before you know it, you will be at the top wondering what got you there."

Choose your wish, plan your route, and take one step at a time.

Understanding what we do and what gives us pleasure changes the energy required to get the reward sought. If you examine what gave you comfort when able and find different ways to get those rewards within your limitations, you will transform your life. You might initially feel frustrated and limited by the constraints put on you by your disability. You will find ways to enable the pleasures and rewards back into your daily life and start enjoying life thoroughly, differently able, despite the limitations imposed upon you.

Nutrition and hydration are two things we must do to live and nurture our bodies. To prevent dehydration, the amount you can build up to is eight 8-ounce glasses per day, which is about 2 litres. Measurements and memory loss, living in the moment, often stop me from drinking the right amount of water. Often I am too tired to drink, and as I lack the body feedback of being thirsty, drinking enough requires me to use a stricter discipline to take in the amount of fluid I need. My caregiver fills two one-litre bottles that I drink during the day. I am a visual person, and doing it this way helps me to see how much I have left to drink for that day. Not everyone likes plain water, but the taste can be varied by adding syrup or steeping a herb tea to sip throughout the day.

Being fully hydrated gives the body the chance to have the water it needs to function at its best. It looks a little time consuming, but every hour I take a drink at least and work my way through it. The reason for drinking pure water is that it only has one essential ingredient, H_2O, and that is easily absorbed. Why not fizzy drinks, you ask? Fizzy drinks usually contain harmful ingredients and enhanced sugars that may interact with your body's best function. I am not saying that you cannot drink whatever you like. I am advocating introducing pure water because then the body absorbs it. It does not have to filter out unsuitable ingredients via the liver and balance the sugar levels it contains, which requires more energy.

I know from experience that with lower energy levels, my body will have less energy for other actions. Fizzy drinks may increase morale or the ability to face your day. However, you may want to consider whether the benefit aligns with your health plan. It's an ongoing balancing of risk and reward.

To feed the body well, you need to eat regularly, perhaps with fewer calories. I requested an appointment with a dietician to establish the number of calories my body consumed daily. She worked out that to keep my weight in check and have all the required nutrients in my diet, I had to work towards a limit of 1500 calories a day. I spent a good few months experimenting with the calorie count of food. If you drink water instead of Coke, you will automatically reduce the calorie content by 139 for every 330ml can of Coca Cola swapped.

You may find it useful to know your basal metabolic rate (BMR). Your BMR is the total number of calories that your body needs to perform basic, life-sustaining functions. You can use an online tool to calculate your personal BMR. You will be asked to input your details, such as age, gender, weight, and height. The calculator will tell you how many calories are needed based on your activity level. If, like me, you use a wheelchair to accessorize your independence, choose the sedentary option for activity, and work out the calories needed. Deduct 250 calories per day to reduce weight slowly. Recalculate monthly as it will change due to weight loss, then plan your daily intake and make changes accordingly.

Each morning I must eat a biscuit to take my medication at breakfast time because some medication cannot be taken on an empty stomach. I used to eat a biscuit that had 60 calories. After researching and reading packets, I found a biscuit with 30 calories. I was able to cut the calorie count without cutting out the cookie. Keep looking at what you eat and evaluate the calories in each meal. To cut down on calories, I also changed the size of my plate. Although I was eating a full plate of food, it was less food. A big plate with a smaller portion and empty areas on your plate would accentuate that you are eating less and might not be viewed in a positive light. When eating out or with family at celebrations, I would eat like everyone else as I certainly did not want to bring attention to myself,

There are two ways of keeping or reducing the weight you have in a wheelchair: eat less or exercise more, and eating less is the easier of the two. If you have the ability and opportunity for exercise, explore the options, and see how you can live best in harmony. Whatever step is necessary to obtain balance, be confident that you can experiment and fine-tune it over time. It requires perseverance, dedication, and willpower, but it is possible.

11

ONE STEP BACK, TWO STEPS FORWARD

There are opportunities even in the most
challenging moments.
— Wangara Maathai

"I have this friend who wants to be a personal
trainer for people with disabilities and thought
you might give her the chance to practice with
you."

My friend's comment seemed as ridiculous as
her encouraging me to climb Mount Everest. The
idea of a personal trainer felt like an insult at the
time. Imagine a middle-aged woman in a
wheelchair, no feeling from the waist down, quite
depressed about being in a wheelchair. She has

lost the ability to walk. The consultant has told her she must prepare herself never to walk again. Couldn't my friend see that I had a hard time being me?

In moments like that, I'm grateful that I have a great sense of humour. My vision of a personal trainer was that guy you find at the gym, barking at you like a drill sergeant to move and go just that little bit farther than comfortable. However, after thinking about her suggestion for a few moments, I realized I had nothing to lose and agreed to work with the trainer as a team.

After six months, the hospital physical therapy I received had come to an end. At the time, I could not move out of the chair unaided, and needed two caregivers and a platform to transfer me. I had no strength at all. Although it was far from my optimum, the impression given was that I had reached an acceptable level. However, they and I were proven wrong.

The personal trainer visited, observed me, and assessed me. She also listened to me. Then after an hour, she proposed coming every week to work with me. *That will be fascinating*, I thought, resisting the urge to roll my eyes. I had never been the gym type, and I didn't fancy myself starting now, but the benefit would be seeing a new human being and moving my body a little.

The first visit came, and the personal trainer and I talked a lot. She examined my perceived limitations and then challenged them. If I said, "I cannot do that," she would encourage me to try. When I said, "I cannot feel the lower half of my body," her answer was, "just because you cannot feel it does not mean it does not work. Even if we detect a tiny muscle movement, we can build it up." At that moment, I gave up my resistance a little. It was perfectly normal to be so tense. My body had suffered significant trauma, and I had to learn to relax and be gentler with myself.

Weeks went by where we talked and moved a little. It was not like my idea of exercise. Still, she encouraged me through movements. From lifting a cup with gradually more liquid content to increase the weight to exploring the moves I needed to be independent as much as possible. We mutually agreed to see how far we could go. There were no limitations. The sky was the limit.

Whenever I would say, "I cannot do that," she would add the word "yet," which changed the proposition. It was not easy by any means, but she worked diligently on the next step. If I could move muscle A, she could strengthen muscle B, which would initiate contact with muscle C, etc. We worked on upper arm strength and then rebuilding my core to enable me to have the power to stand up more comfortably with the turning platform. It seemed endless, but I could sense some progress, and although I did not believe in myself, she believed in me, and that was a great comfort.

Time after time, she would show me that even if I said I could not do something, I could do it after a few months. If I phoned her to tell her I was having a bad day, she would still come and work with me. The secret was a willingness to show up. I have no idea how she came to be in my life at the right moment, but she had. She may have looked more like a member of the Hells Angels, fierce and determined, but she came to help me.

It took a year for me to grasp that I was making slow progress in my mobility. Our bodies retreat and tense up when we suffer trauma, keeping our core and vital organs safe. It is an instinctual response. The flaw is that we continue this tactic far beyond the impact moment, and we must relearn and adjust to our bodies, our safe space, and who we genuinely are.

One area we shy away from talking about is the damage done to our internal organs. Spinal cord

damage does not exclude injury to any part of the
body that the spinal cord facilitates. In my case, it
also affected my bladder and bowels. That
annoyed me more than anything else because
being clean and dry is an essential milestone in
our childhood. Losing it takes us right back to
those feelings of embarrassment and discomfort.
Eventually, I could no longer perform bodily
functions consciously. It would require
intervention, and it caused me a great deal of
anguish.

Based on the facts, the doctors investigate
whether the body will repair itself. Please do not
be embarrassed. It will get better. Medical science
has reached such levels that many treatments for
malfunctions are mechanical. It does mean more
equipment in general, but it becomes part of who
you are and is eventually accepted by you. It
becomes liberating. I was apprehensive about it all
until my son explained that some functions
happening in the conscious environment have an
underlying mechanism of still occurring without
awareness.

Babies are not born with the ability to be clean
and know when they need to relieve themselves.
Still, their bodies carry on regardless to perform
those functions. It is a bit of a journey to get used

to having a catheter and not be self-conscious about it. Still, when it works, it offers strategic advantages. You will never be caught short without toilet facilities, etc. It took some getting used to thinking it was too visible. Still, a catheter is preferable to not having one and being exposed to skin damage and bedsores, which are more dangerous. Applying risk and reward, you will find that having a catheter turns into a bonus as the risks of not having one is more hazardous and uncomfortable.

The nurse who initially broached the subject with me was using the words that formed part of her daily vocabulary. I cringed a lot and had no idea how to express myself and my dilemma adequately. It is not a subject we talk about as adults. I was nervous, and what seemed reasonable to her was alien and uncomfortable to me. I need not have been so tense. It was a part of her daily vocabulary and, as such, quite usual to discuss. I did have conversations with others in the hospital who had gone through the procedure, explaining how better their life quality was with a catheter. It became easier to discuss.

Years later, my elderly father had the same issue but found it extremely hard to talk about for the same reasons. He was beating himself up about the fact that his body was cancelling out his bodily functions. When I told him it was sad but typical, and there were solutions available, he relaxed a little. These conversations would make this experience less painful to deal with. He did not feel he could talk about such subjects easily. It happens to be the most visited topic with caregivers. Please relax. There will be many feelings and thoughts about this subject. Explore each one with curiosity and talk with the health professionals in your team. They will find a long-lasting solution that works for you and your lifestyle.

Eventually, they fitted me with a suprapubic catheter, which is inserted into the bladder through a cut in the tummy, a few inches below the navel. As my bed got wheeled to the technician's workroom where the procedure would take place, I remembered a dream I had the day before. I dreamt that he was going to attack me with a giant knitting needle. I suppose you could call it a Freudian slip of sorts as I am a keen knitter. We talked and joked, but as I had no idea what they were about to do, I asked, and he produced this implement that looked as tall as a knitting needle. I was calm, and the experience was akin to having your ears pierced. A momentary shock, yes, but all over in a flash. And then, instant relief.

A catheter needs maintenance and to be replaced at regular intervals. It is carried out expertly by district nurses who visit me at home. Replacing a suprapubic catheter is routine now after nine years. It has been a journey with the flexibility of timing to replace it. Overall, the replacement of a catheter by a skilled nurse takes minutes. You think you might never get used to it. It needs a few hours to settle down, but you will mostly have no awareness of it. Catheters do increase the risk of urinary tract infections (UTI). Still, after having one, you will be more vigilant and know the symptoms. In my case, I become a nasty old hag who criticizes everyone near and dear.

Miners used to have a caged canary in the mines to alert them to dangerous gasses being present. My husband is my canary. He puts up with some of it and then suggests, "Should we get your urine tested?" He has been right every time so far. I only once had a severe UTI, which affected my perception of reality. I convinced myself certain events had happened, and yet they only happened in my awareness. That UTI affected my mental health and was a scary experience. That was an embarrassing moment to get over. But I did get over it and continued to be me and act like me, not the nasty old hag.

A UTI affects each of us differently. The doctors treat it efficiently with a course of antibiotics in my case. The reward of having a catheter does mitigate the embarrassment of not having one for sure. The medical team will introduce this subject as sensitively as possible, and you will find a way to navigate this territory too. The medical team is knowledgeable, and the only action required is to face the embarrassment you feel—something you might need time to process. The road to some recovery and finding your harmony is sometimes long in time and individual experience. Take the time to relax and ponder. On such occasions, I ask myself, this or better: can I tolerate it, or is there a better solution for this?

When you get home, the aim will be to recover and heal to your optimum in a safe environment. By now, your journal should have many aspects you want to improve or change. The most crucial element for your journaling is to find why you want to heal and why you want to live your life the way you envisage it. My 'why' is to continue to be available to my children and support them. Your why may be different. And when you have thought about that and defined it, you can start by making changes one day at a time, one thought at a time, one action at a time, one habit at a time, one change at a time.

You will build resilience and work towards your defined goals one baby step at a time. Armed with your why and your plan, you can start implementing small actions that will provide feedback and upon which you can build to reach your goals. You will find that tiny window of opportunity that allows you to haul yourself out of your imposed chrysalis and take flight. Remember, it is a dangerous process, vulnerable, exhausting, and will seem never-ending. One day you will get there. Rest if you must, but never give up.

The aim of being home firstly is to try and stay out of the hospital needing immediate care. Changes to routine, changes to nutrition, changes to timing, changes to everything will influence and cause upset constantly. Every time I came home from the hospital, I would feel less capable than in the hospital. Each time I would need an extra day to accept changes in my routine. To stop overwhelm and panic, know that you have everything that you need to stabilize being at home. Care professionals will have considered your care needs, and you will have most things at hand to maintain your healing progress at home. Be gentle with yourself.

What helps is to set out those areas for which you can control the outcome against those you cannot control. My mind works in scientific ways, looking at differences, and making decisions based on the data. I did not respond well to my pre-injury bed coming home. It was replaced with one that was as close to a hospital bed as possible. The physiotherapist knew I could cope with a similar bed, which ensured I would get as good a rest as in the hospital. I may not have liked the idea, but I did not have to like it. It just was the best option for me, and I had to adapt to it. After all, sleep and rest are vital to recovery.

My routine consisted of getting up, getting washed and dressed, breakfast, and staying awake in my wheelchair. To make it through the day, which ended at 8 p.m., I required rest after lunch. It was far from what I wanted to do, feeling like a kid, but I needed to rest to continue my recovery. At least when you sleep 50 percent of your day or more, time flies.

The breathing techniques and meditation underpinned the rest and recovery process. Breathing and meditation balanced my being. At that moment, there are no expectations of doing anything, just moments of being. I could listen to audiobooks to entertain my brain and learn.

You will often progress three stages on your plan then revert by two. I understand how exasperating that can be. I would sometimes catch an infection or need some medical intervention, and for months I would alternate between living at home and back in the hospital. Still, staying stable is staying one step ahead. If you feel frustrated because this seems to be taking ages and is such slow progress, stay focused.

Your frustration may seem unbearable at times, yet by following a constant supporting routine (breathing, meditation, journaling, audiobooks, and much rest), it will pass, and you will return home. The data will provide proof that the time spans between returning to the hospital or staying home become more prolonged, and time will lengthen between having to go back into hospital and managing at home.

Whenever you get sent back to the hospital, you may feel fearful and discouraged. You will know when you are afraid because you will feel it and face it. You will find ways to become calmer and reassured by medical attention and find your inner calm. The other one, discouragement, is far more subtle. It attaches itself to you without being visible. It chips away at you consistently with questions like Will I ever get better? Will I work again? Will I walk again? When will this stop? Who cares? You may come to feel incredibly low and lonely and feel no one in the world knows what you are going through, and no one understands you. I am here to tell you that I know. I am standing with you, and so is your God, to accompany you on this journey.

The solution to overcome discouragement is to find the courage to persevere. After two years in the hospital, I wondered whether I would ever get to go back to my familiar surroundings, to my family, and my beloved garden. At one point, I thought it would never happen, and discouragement had crept into my awareness and taken over. The encouraging words spoken by my personal trainer were so powerful: "Just because you cannot feel your muscles moving, does not automatically mean they don't work." You must test the question and record your answer. Just because it does or does not happen one time, you must persevere over a while and test out those limitations. Never give up.

Are the tremors real? Is there a millimetre of difference? If all the perseverance brings you the same result repeatedly, then yes, consider the loss of it temporarily and give it another shot a little later. If there is a flicker of change, a flash of movement, you can work with it and persevere. Revisit that movement from time to time as, like a flowing river, change is constant. Sometimes you need one muscle to function to combine with another. It's painfully slow and requires perseverance. Is it easy? No, it's not easy. However, if every day you build in a little step to take you there and follow through with it, you might be surprised as to what happens.

I was depressed at the prospect of not being able to walk and hike in the countryside, of course. When I considered doing that, I was unable to stand, balance, or move. It was impossible even to visualize. If the expected outcome of your injury is that you will never walk again, as in my story, define what a walk means to you. If it means a hike up a mountain, then maybe not. If walking is as in walking around the house, then perhaps. Suppose it meant getting out of bed, standing up, and transferring to your wheelchair. More probable? Yes. It's called reframing your expectations.

To me, the word impossible means I am possible. I want to be at the top of the staircase, but if I look at the stairs, I will be discouraged and maybe feel it's just not worth it. It will look unattainable and too hard. Do not go there. I am here to encourage you to look at the one step in front of you. I want to help you to concentrate and focus on managing that one step, whatever comes next. When you conquer that one step, you will rejoice and still not look at the staircase. You will see the next level and figure out how you will tackle that one. How do you eat an elephant? One bite at a time. How do you solve an enormous challenge? One step at a time.

Here is what I discovered by chance. It appears runners who win the race quite often prepare themselves by running the race virtually. They see the landscape, and they run the almost whole course of the competition in preparation. They practically manage to breathe at the right moment, hydrate at the right moment and opportunity. They virtually lean into the bend, and with determination, they pass the finish line. They do not just focus on the finish line because that will slow them up towards the end. They focus past the finishing line keeping their goal in mind of winning the race and keep running.

Dreams feel very real. The body does not know the difference between an actual experience and a virtual one. Practice your next step in your virtual perception, and your body will react as if you had just performed that action. Build in a virtual workout. You can persevere by doing exercises virtually until you feel strong enough to implement them for real.

12

PARALLEL DIMENSIONS

We must not, in trying to think about how we can make a big difference, ignore the small daily differences we can make which, over time, add up to big differences that we often cannot foresee.
— Marian Wright Edelman

I enjoy my virtual life. When I cannot go out and experience something physically, I live the experience virtually and get some of the same endorphins to flood my body. Who needs to drive a Porsche? You could just imagine driving it, feeling the wind whip up your hair, until you can do it for real.

This year (2020) COVID-19 grounded everyone

and put us all under house arrest. Despite being locked in my house for sixteen weeks, it was to be a fabulous time. Many events went virtual, including all the festivals I was interested in, enabling me to participate on my computer without being there physically. I ticked off a few experiences from my bucket list by visiting various wool festivals and the famous virtual Chelsea Flower Show. I could not smell the roses, but I could admire the many garden designs that made my heart sing.

The way to be is different. Instead of looking way ahead into the future, we can change that scenario to wake up and show up. Each day I greet the world and am thankful I slept well and rested. I say hello to the world, check my health, and say I need to take a step today.

Your secret tool is the journal. Your secret weapon is perseverance and the courage to tackle one tiny step repeatedly. You just must show up ready to go every day. Your journal will inform you of what to look forward to that day. You have something to offer the world, and you need to believe in your ability to do that.

I send cards from my phone, so my friends and family get congratulatory messages just like I would tell them when meeting them next in person. I get the same pleasure, and they get the same expression of love and friendship, but it is created with the resources I have. It is the same action performed much slower and different than usual. The feeling and joy I get from the interaction are the same.

If you have a dream, what steps can you take today towards that dream to bring it into your reality? As you take that one step with perseverance, you will be one step closer. Take control of your thoughts, write down the goals in your journal, and plan small steps towards the impossible. Or use dictation to record your words if writing is more challenging.

Discouragement does not thrive on fear, but on our hesitancy to be who we visualize we are. Take the steps necessary to get there in time. Safely. Dream big. Know who you are, and challenge those little obstacles by breaking them down. Persevere in doing all you can with the resources you have to achieve the outcome you set for yourself in your visualization. Write them down, record them on your phone, compare your progress, and find creative solutions to get the result you need.

Take James, for example, who I met in the cottage hospital. When he went home, he was not able to use his hands. How was he going to keep busy, watch films, and engage with life? As it turns out, his voice can control his action commands. That meant that by having a voice-controlled TV, he can scroll, choose what he wants to watch, adjust the volume, and even record his favourite TV programs.

Where he thought he would be helpless, he can manage those functions, not with his hands but with his voice. What he thought was impossible and led to frustration and discouragement has changed his life by following through. He can watch TV, change channels, record programs, not as we think he would. James is confidently showing those around him that he is differently able and that anything is possible. He is just achieving outcomes in a different and unexpected way. It took a good while to practice and get right. Still, with research and practice, he is now awesome at finding his way around the home entertainment system in his home environment without any help.

Anything is possible. It is important to note that there is a distinction between possibility and likelihood. If you interpret possibility as likelihood, that implies it will happen automatically. Possibility requires constant effort and perseverance. There are no guarantees, but I don't want you to give up before you have explored all possibilities.

The time spent so far on recovery and writing in your journal may crystallize your thoughts about what you need to be at your optimum, not necessarily on what you want. In my experience, I never got what I wanted until I had satisfied what I needed to stay healthy. The primary need is to look after our bodies and our mental health, and that will look different for every person.

To create a baseline means to note down all the things that are going well when you are stable. Whether you have slept the usual eight hours soundly or interrupted. Whether your digestion and elimination are working seamlessly or whether your temperature is above average, etc. In the hospital, your temperature, blood pressure, and blood sugars are checked regularly to spot the first signs of difference. For the most part, you are doing the same at home. I learned that every time I ate a particular substance, my liver got overloaded as it was working overtime to process vital medication. Eating that food seemed just to push it over the limit.

I reached a point where I finally thought I had cracked it. I was not going to the hospital frequently and getting used to being in my home environment. The frustration was still high, and I learned that the simple fact of being emotional, whether frustrated or excited, took its toll. I had to learn through meditation to notice the emotion and either let it go or accept the consequences of its effects. Great when you are happy, but less exciting when the emotion is anger or frustration. My standard response would be "that's nice" or "I see that," but I needed to learn to let go of the anger, frustration, excitement, and find a happy bubble to exist in. Why not try it the next time you feel anger and frustration or any negative feeling bubbling up? Get into that meditative state and think, "that's a frustration for you."

I must have made a wish some years before to stay in bed for as long as I could, with room service. Guess what? That had come to fruition. Maybe not how I imagined it, but the essence of it was. Indeed, you are okay resting in that bed while some major body restructuring is going on. Every moment you can observe what is happening will inform the next step to take.

There is a risk and a reward for everything. An 18-year-old discovers that alcohol can lead to a high and drinks often. A 35-year-old may not drink as much because of the risk of a hangover. A hangover affects life the next day and is usually less pleasant than the reward of being drunk and disorderly. He will then drink less often.

Just because you can do something does not mean you have to do it. I can make a cup of tea even though it takes twenty minutes now to achieve. The reward of making that cup of tea is appropriate if I am desperately in need of it, and there is no one available to help me get it. The risk is that it demands twenty minutes of my time and energy. It means manoeuvring the wheelchair back and forth several times. I need to be incredibly careful not to be unsteady with a hot cup of tea in a sealed travel cup. The effort spent making that cup of tea means I will have lost that energy portion to do something I enjoy more that day. A choice must be made continuously as to risk and reward. You will get to make choices to find a balance between what you must do and relinquish some of those tasks to get to do fun stuff you want to do.

I choose to eat light most of the time at home, which rewards me with less unpleasant symptoms. The monthly blood tests come back within acceptable ranges. However, when I go out, which is a deliberate activity, or someone brings me a piece of their "death by chocolate" birthday cake, I have choices. I do not say no to eating it. Although I know it will cause symptoms, I eat a small piece and share my friend's birthday celebration. The friend does not care how much cake I eat but might be sad if I said, "Thanks, but I cannot eat that!"

Priorities change. My health took the number one place, followed by being a mum to my four children and a wife to my husband. The circle then widened, and because I took care of my needs first, I did have some energy for my wants. In the past, I travelled the world but probably did not fully appreciate that I could visit or even take in the beauty of those places. I felt I needed to do things, yet I neglected my needs.

We need oxygen (breathing), hydration (water), and nutrition. These essentials will take us to a place of optimum health where our bodies can rebuild and strengthen through rest and exercise. When we reach that place, we can fulfil other needs that feed us, inspire us, and help us grow. When it all falls into place, we can feel happy despite a spinal injury, a job, and find our voice or virtual voice to express the person we are. We have a body, but we also have a soul. When the body functions just a little differently, we can still be authentic. Your journal should help you envisage how to express your authentic self into the world.

This moment is an opportunity to reset your life. It is not the easiest of roads to go down, but it will open your eyes. It will help you see and give energy to what matters most. You will be able to make decisions based on what you have discovered to be your authentic self. You will make changes.

You will often consider "what if" scenarios. What if I was not in a wheelchair? What if I was not disabled? These scenarios focus your mind on the past or project your attention to the future. I've learned to be in the moment. The only commitment I made every morning was to be grateful for waking up, thankful for the care I received, and focus on whatever activity was in the present.

Being in the present takes away the trauma of what happened to get to this present moment. Thinking about how far you would like to go with your health may be too painful to think about compared to where you are now. The past is too traumatic, the future uncertain, and the only place to live is now. Sometimes now is hard also, but little moments are easier to tolerate and eventually pass.

13

BASELINE DECISIONS

Start where you are. Use what you have. Do
what you can.
— Arthur Ashe

Imagine a tree under which are three creatures, a
monkey, a bird, and a giraffe. The first task given to
the three animals is to touch the highest branch.
The winner is the bird, as it was the quickest to get
up there. The second task was to climb the tree.
The monkey won as neither the bird nor the
giraffe can climb. The third task was to eat some
leaves. The giraffe won that one. With his long
neck, his head was right next to the leaves. All
three animals won an aspect of achieving a task
but could not win at all three. Yet if we consider

the winner to be the one with the highest score, none of them pass one.

"Disabled" is a term given by able-bodied people to other people they consider unable to do the same actions as them in the same way. If I am to achieve the identical goal as them in the same way they are, then, of course, I am going to fail sometimes. A giraffe is never going to climb a tree, and the monkey is not going to fly as we understand it. If I just look at the end goal, I might find a different way to achieve that goal using different elements. One does not exclude the other, and there is enough room in the world for everyone to work out what works best.

You can represent a differently able person by choice, whether those choices be big or small. The most critical difference in decision making is that before my injury, I would take a risk because the drawbacks and consequences would be easy to overcome. However, when you have health issues, there are more things to consider.

At our 25th wedding anniversary, my son organized a meal in a rather pricey setting. On the day of, probably noticing the "disabled guest note," the resaurant phoned to say there were stairs to get to the dining room. They suggested strong men carry me across the dining room to the table. I had visions of being carried by footmen like royalty in a sedan chair. Those visions quickly morphed into the dreadful image of me being bumped about awkwardly like a spectacle. I felt horrified as I did not want to draw attention to myself, and it posed a safety issue.

My husband enjoys a glass of wine. So he could party, we arranged for my youngest son to drive and take us all safely home. He did not have any alcohol because he took responsibility to get us back in one piece. At the meal, I had a thimble of wine. I thought, why not? We are celebrating. Bear in mind, I am not supposed to have alcohol with my medication, but I thought a thimble would be okay. It was not. It upset my balance, and my son had to keep the walker steady to ensure my safety while transferring into the car.

All of that could have been avoided by sticking to no alcohol. That day I learned that no alcohol means no alcohol. Even a small overstepping of the boundaries set adversely affected my transfers in an out of the car. Nothing we could not overcome, yet something I wish I had thought about with a little more care.

Divas can do anything stating conditions. They usually say, "Yes, I can do that performance; however, my dressing room always has a vase with fifteen red roses. And I do not drink water darling, only champagne." Hence, when the diva performs, it is entirely the norm to find a vase with fifteen (not sixteen) red roses, and a bottle of champagne in her dressing room.

It won't be the same for you, but do cultivate your inner diva or divo. What are your ideal requirements for daily living? To "perform," the right conditions must be met. What temperature are you most comfortable at while you do not move. Instead of heating the whole house in winter to a higher temperature for me, which was uncomfortable for the other housemates, I discovered a system that would individually control each radiator. That way, the room I spent most of my time in could be warmer than the rest of the house, and everyone seemed happy. The internet offers different options and considerations for everything in an instant.

Visiting a friend might be possible but not if the friend lives on the 4th floor of a house and there is no lift. If this situation presents itself, why not think creatively and turn it around? You may find it too challenging to meet in that location. Don't give up on the visit but consider changing to a place that fits your needs. A cafe has outdoor seating on level ground. You can rock up in your wheelchair. You can share a coffee and chat and have the same benefits as visiting elsewhere. It is a bit different, but the essence of the visit is the same.

Go back to baseline. When you have noted down the norm for feeling at your best, you can try things and compare the outcome. If I stop eating and cease my normal activities, there is the possibility that something else will demand attention in my body. I then need time to check all data against the baseline and seek medical advice if required. We don't win or lose; we win or learn and adapt.

There could be other things to notice. When I am at a lower level of health, I cannot stop talking, but give a running commentary on what my caregiver needs to do next. I micromanage, which is very irritating, as she has been doing this job daily for nearly five years. It is my way of controlling my immediate surroundings when my health is out of control. Then we can signpost infections with the doctor before they become unmanageable. It is very irritating for my housemates, but they are now aware of that signpost and gently question what is going on.

The process of making decisions based on risk and reward takes time and a lot of trial and error.

But it will help you to stay stable and at baseline instead of peaks and troughs in your health management. You will suddenly get it and feel a lot more able to face your day.

I have regular blood tests that inform my medical team about how my body performs and that it is stable. However, if the data is outside set criteria, they make changes to my medication to get it back to the medical baseline. At the same time, I evaluate what could have changed that data. Was it eating a lot of a certain kind of food, or maybe cutting down on sleep to watch a movie? Often you may not have control over how your body reacts and feel disabled by your condition; however, you do control your daily activities. You can choose to change activities and take different actions so that the worst impact is avoided.

Do not let anyone's perception of you define you. Many able people see a disabled person as struggling in a wheelchair, whereas your understanding may be different. Comments such as "such a shame you have ended up in a wheelchair" are met by me counteracting that my wheelchair is a bike. Far from disabling me, it enables me to get around. It may be slower, but without it, I would be in a different predicament. That usually is not a reaction they expect.

Most people do not have the experience of how being pushed in a wheelchair feels and affects you. Nurses and caregivers have that simulation as part of their training. They know how disempowering it feels when you have no control over where you are going, at which speed, etc. My scariest experience was my children wheeling me about in Disneyland. They thought it would be fun to change the direction of the wheelchair quickly and sway crazily. They were playing, and that was understandable. All the while, I was so uncomfortable and dizzy without them having a clue.

We are all different. And on occasions, we don't voice what the experience was like for us because we are not aware we can express it. We do not want to complain. We feel uncomfortable. Try to use your voice in a graceful way to help the other person understand how the situation affected you and how together you can make it better next time. Compromising is a new skill to practice.

I am also a diabetic, but I have a sweet tooth. After every phone session with my therapist, I would ask my caregiver to make me a cup of hot chocolate (complete with cream and marshmallows). I would request a sticky bun, which was total sugar overload. It would result in a spike on my blood sugar monitor, followed by unpleasant feelings. I finally understood that becoming emotional resulted in a sugar craving. At best, I would change the sticky bun to an apple with great crunch potential and a glass of mint tea —both healthier options, still sweet but not near the sugar overload. The risk of eating less healthy food to be comforted was diminished by eating food that had a lower negative impact on my blood sugar levels. Of course, there are occasions where a day is needed without the usual constraints present. If you follow a diet every day, you need to let go every now and then to stay the course. The same goes for perceived limitations. Build in a crazy day where you have just a little too much fun but follow that with a rest day later.

Keeping data and writing down what fuel we add to our bodies, moods, and how our bodies react provides valuable information. We can then better understand the impact of those things on overstretched body systems. We all have different resources. I am trying to encourage you to see further than the difficulties that present themselves.

When I was a young girl, my parents would buy cards with paintings made by artists with no limbs. I questioned how they managed to paint such beautiful pictures and discovered they painted using their mouth to hold the paintbrush. Some even painted with their toes. Far from me, concentrating on how strange that was, I was in awe. They had the tenacity to paint and overcome obstacles using different resources they had available. You can do that too. Over time, I wish you could explore the world. Take what it has to offer you instead of having the perspective that you cannot do anything because of your circumstances. I believe in you.

Please do not let anyone's perception of you define who you are or what you are capable of. Only you can test those boundaries safely and create your path to fulfil your potential. It is a leap of faith at this moment in time. Still, I am encouraging you from the other side to show you that anything is possible. Your expression and vision of you are still possible yet different from what you have experienced so far. You will emerge as a butterfly.

14

NURTURING MOTIVATION

Whether you think you can or you think you can't, you're right.
— Henry Ford

Aesop's fable of the tortoise and the hare is the story of difference. The hare and the tortoise undertake the race. A common perspective shows that the hare will win the race being much faster. However, the tortoise wins the race to the astonishment of collective perception. The hare decided to rest and was overtaken by the tortoise, which continued the course, calmly, slowly, and steadily. The tortoise did not quit at the beginning of the race, holding on to the common perception that the hare was faster and would outrun him. He had other qualities and approaches to the competition. I changed from the hare into the tortoise. It may take more time and effort to get where I want to be. However, slow and steady wins the race. Let's go. You can and will do it if you believe you can. The choice is yours.

Being as healthy as possible will bring you the foundation upon which to build your unique contribution to the world. Take time to process that thought. Reread it, absorb it afresh. Whatever changed your appearance and functioning means you will not be able to pursue your potential with the resources you had. You have lost some support, but there are others you have not yet explored or invented. Find that optimism, that hunger for life. Instead of attempting actions too fast and furious, go slow and steady as that will ultimately win the race in the end.

Whenever a closed-door presents itself in your life, I want to encourage you to look for a window. It could become a window of opportunity. I experienced that by paying attention to a different aspect of my being, and I would do my best to enjoy that. It would ultimately change the situation. Although I often could not change the physical outcome of something, such as pain somewhere, I would concentrate on making my

body as comfortable as possible, retreat into
meditation, or listen to a session of yoga nidra.
After a while, I would not be so tense, and the pain
would be breathed through and thanked for
showing me something was not right.

Instead of fighting your body with your mind, I
would encourage you to work with it. Give it
additional resources and find the window of
opportunity. Rest if you must, but never give up.

You are a beautiful complex whole human
being made up of parts. Some parts will respond
better than others. Each one connects as a part of
the whole. Where my eyesight diminished, my
capacity to hear would increase and compensate.
Some taste buds would disappear, and I would
cultivate a more distinguished palette and
concentrate on the texture of the food. We can find
pleasure in a different area of experience. It is not
about staring at the closed door but looking for
the window, never giving up, and looking for the
gap safely.

I am confident that providing your body with
elements that will build strength and not
aggravate the physical body will give it features to
strengthen the body. I use care products without
harmful chemicals to reduce the impact of
additional substances on a sensitive body. The

reason I drink plant-based milk instead of cow's milk is that I tolerate it far better. It is still milk, but not as traditionally thought of.

When my weight increased as a result of not moving as much and the impact of the medications I took, I had limited choices. Could I exercise more? Could I eat less? What could I do in terms of exercise? I built in a little activity into the garden daily, pushing the wheels of my wheelchair manually. At the same time, I established the number of calories my body needed daily by asking to see a dietician. Armed with the information, I need to limit my intake to a maximum of 1500 calories per day. I started to experiment to get the most nutrition out of that allowance.

Reducing the calories to an arbitrary figure is not the point. Your body needs a certain number of calories to stay healthy and repair itself where required. I found out I could substitute foods with a lower calorie count, which left me enough to eat some of the foods that gave me pleasure. I replaced my large dinner plate with a smaller plate, which would still look full of delicious food. I concentrated on abundance and not the lack of food.

If your body craves a particular food, you can

NURTURING MOTIVATION   151

decide to give in to that on occasion. The different meal plan is in existence when you are at home. Meeting friends for a meal out, you can make informed choices on the menu in line with your abilities. A mistake I made often was to choose pizza and then take an awkward fifteen minutes to cut the thing. At the same time, my friends looked on at my awkwardness, my difficulty, and frustration. They wanted to help yet not draw attention to the issue. I progressed to asking the waiter to cut my pizza with a pizza cutter, which they always do no questions asked. You may increase your feeling of not being able to do something able people take for granted simply because you do not feel ready to ask. In practice, most restaurants and venues will be happy to help you in a way that does not call for special attention.

After my stroke, I couldn't cut my food. It was too embarrassing for me to try and struggle while the others ate their meal. I finally built up the courage to ask whether they would be able to cut my food into bite sizes in the kitchen, and they usually obliged. The situation meant I could start eating at the same time as most people around the table. We do this for our children when they have difficulty, but we are afraid to speak up when this simply would make the occasion more pleasurable. If you need a bigger cup to drink out of, instead of a china cup, ask for a mug. Let people know what you need to complete the action to be differently able.

My most painful activity is filling in welfare benefit forms that need you to specify all the things you cannot do and need help with. Get a friend to fill in the forms with you. That way, you won't use up energy to complete them. It gets super emotional and drains your energy. Personally, when you tell me that I cannot do something, my inner rebel comes out fighting with both fists, stomping on the ground, mad like hell. I shout, *you just watch me!*

I do not accept the limitations put on me by others, but I strive to test how far I can go with that. My dad quite often used to tell me, "That's too complicated for your age. You will not be able to do that." It made me angry, and I tried even harder to achieve the outcome. Being told I could not do something to me was a motivator. Whenever someone says you cannot do something, test it out in your safe environment. Don't just assume you cannot do something based on someone else's limitations imposed on you.

To actively change things in your life, I want

you to pay attention to the words you speak and others use when talking to you. I heard, "you will never walk again," which caused me an immense sadness. I spent every day mourning the things I could no longer do, and it was affecting my motivation. I could not try harder to improve the things I could do, and one day I decided to reframe my negative thoughts to positive ones actively. I would work out how to do something. I was determined to concentrate on the things I could do and not the ones I could no longer manage in my eyes or the eyes of others.

Grow in confidence instead of approaching the situation as a dependent disabled person. See the person inside first, the authentic person you are, the unique mixture of talents and perseverance. Try as much as is comfortable, and if you need help, please voice the question. It is a process, but the more tasks you can comfortably and safely participate in, the more empowered you will feel. The more the balance will shift from seeing yourself as disabled and become differently able.

15

LASTING IMPRESSIONS

For lots of us, disabled people are not our
teachers or our doctors or our manicurists.
We're not real people. We are there to inspire.
And in fact, I am sitting on this stage looking
like I do in this wheelchair, and you are
probably kind of expecting me to inspire you.
— Stella Young

When you suffer a traumatic spinal injury, you
will need time to physically heal from that
moment. The physical healing will often be
quicker and more logical than facing the
psychological impact of the injury. You suddenly
stop being the person you were, expressing your
individuality, feeling you have lost a vital part of

yourself. You have indeed lost some functions and cannot express who you are in the way most people take for granted, but the individual person you are is very much intact. If you explore how you can express and do things differently, you might find the window of opportunity where before you saw a closed door.

Most of us go through a period of mental blah, followed by anxiety and panic. In time we count our blessings. Next, we find the value of our family support. If you are secure in your family, be grateful for your foundation. If you do not have family support, find a friend who will take the path by your side. You need someone with you to take that path, someone who knows you and can provide an able perspective on your questions. Then you can compare the responses and test within safe boundaries what options there are. I cannot be taken out by certain friends because they are not strong enough to push me. I must also be mindful of their abilities when planning an outing and consider the right circumstances for everyone involved. If I am considerate of their needs, they will more than likely be thinking about mine.

Find out next what direction you go in. Why did you do what you did professionally? What motivated you to do what you were doing? What is your passion? Why do you keep going? For me, it was the wish to continue to be the mother of my children. I wanted to be part of their lives, and I did not necessarily want them to see me struggle visibly. I was not capable of fulfilling all the roles I had played in my life before the injury. There were so many of them, and I needed to return to basics. Making a cake for a fundraiser was no longer possible. Was there another way to contribute? Could I manage selling tickets or taking phone calls and feel included?

What follows is a practical activity to undertake with your support partner. Once you have your 'why,' I would like you to try and reframe your thoughts. Find a piece of paper and draw a vertical line in the middle. If that is difficult, ask your support partner to do everything or help you do the exercise within your abilities. On the left-hand side of the paper, list or dictate all the things you are not able to do. I could no longer read books due to bad eyesight and I found holding a book and turning the page very difficult. On my list, on the left side of the paper, my husband (who is my support partner) wrote, *I cannot read a book*. All the other things I could not do were listed on that piece of paper. The list was rather depressing, and I cried real tears when he wrote those things down. Seeing them on paper somehow made them more present. But this is the point at which reframing my thoughts began. On the right side of the paper, I dictated the same sentence to him as a reframed possibility without the negative: *I enjoy reading books.*

Once you get all the things you cannot do on a piece of paper, you can look at the items in the left-hand column, brainstorm, and then work out how to do them differently. Your brain will rest and find solutions you could have never found immediately. One of the "cannot do" items on my list was: *I can't get in touch with the children.* That reframed as: *I get in touch with the children with ease, and we talk honestly.* That was made possible with the use of a smartphone. Each of my children already had smartphones, and although I had never taken part in communicating virtually, this seemed to be an opportunity and a different avenue to follow. While I was still in the hospital, my husband asked one of my sons to acquire a smartphone with more options and functions, which allowed the children to ask me anything that way.

Initially, I did manage just to take a call, and when I transferred to a single room was able to flick the smartphone to speakerphone when they called. Next, I had to learn to use the keyboard to text them. It took a couple of weeks for one of them to suggest I did not have to spell all the words out. That advice made me feel the generation gap, but at least it made texting much quicker. I could dictate my messages using the microphone. Generally, communicating with them was fun and positive. The smartphone held my music and audiobooks as well as general information and data. Using face recognition technology reduces the mental energy required to memorize passwords and login details. It also provides a safe and independent way to access some functions.

My husband, who until then had visited me daily, changed some visits to phone conversations, which were a welcome relief after he had worked all day. My existence gradually changed from seeing people in their physical presence to having human contact using technology. It is not the same as meeting face to face in the same room, but it comes a close second. In the future, maybe it will be standard procedure to conduct medical appointments virtually to discuss our medical treatments. That would cut out the mammoth efforts and save the energy required to get transported to those appointments. It would enable us to speak from a position of equality using the same tools. A physical trip would then only be required if urgent attention was needed.

The adapted home environment facilitated my care, not just care at home. It established a new way to express myself to the world and join in (or not) as I preferred at the time. I grew my virtual presence.

Did you know the fire department offers a free home consultation visit that informs you of how to build a safe environment in case of an emergency? That visit resulted not only in making my room safe from smoke (should we have a fire), but it also provided them with details about my disability. They would know exactly where to locate and evacuate me from the property in the most appropriate manner. Being in a bed with raised sides, unable to get out, created a fear of being roasted alive. The fire brigade, knowing the building layout and the limitations of my disability, would have the information required to do their best work in case of an emergency. Many utility firms have a priority register where they can account for your disability status and requirements in case of emergencies. Not having access to electricity and water would make life so much more challenging. Even telephone companies can have a direct number for you to get in touch. It makes communication and actions less traumatic for people with disabilities. Explore what is available to build peace of mind.

After settling at home, changing a few things, and accepting some changes to my routine, I was ready to leave my safe bubble and venture outside. Not that cabin fever was an issue, but I felt I needed to explore the outside world a little further. For that to happen, I would need to explore the options available for my wheelchair, build more muscles, and venture out small distances in fair weather. Rain makes it just a bit harder. It rains regularly here, and that can make planning and disappointment an exercise. It takes months to get to a level where going out is possible. Persevere, take little steps, and see how far it takes you.

Another loss was not being able to go on holiday. At least that's what I thought until a friend suggested, "If you cannot visit X, let X come to you." There are a variety of online resources available via Google, museums, zoos, national parks, festivals, etc. Whatever your interest, you will find virtual sources online. You can study for a qualification online. I am a fan of fibre events and have found classes online that I would never be able to take physically part in easily. I managed with a week prior and after to take part in my parents' 60th wedding anniversary and my son's graduation. It took a precise operation plan to prepare for the events, but I attended them and I'm glad I did. My perseverance paid off. It is not possible until you have faced the impossible.

Identify different options when achieving a goal is too difficult. See if there is a way to achieve the same outcome in a different way. For example, I love cooking, and most recipes ask you to sauté small pieces of an onion as the base for the sauce. Cutting an onion is a nightmare for me and also unsafe. How else can I get the pieces of onion for my recipe together? I could ask my helper to cut an onion and set it aside until I needed it later. Or, as I really want to be independent-identified, I could purchase a bag of ready-cut frozen onions. Who knew?

To attend a three-hour event included fourteen days just thinking about how I would travel, where I would stay, what I would wear, how to achieve the outcome safely, etc. I do most activities with a balance of time and energy. Some activities can be visited by video link too when you explain the difficulty you have in attending. We all have different dreams and aspirations, but gently and slowly work out your step at your speed and move forward.

Planning in this way becomes your very own adventure. You can work on your plan every day, and when the time is right, you will be able to go on the adventure well prepared and ready to give it your best shot. You will get the benefit and the result you planned. And what if you are not ready within the timeline you set yourself? That is a disappointment, of course, but it does not mean you will never achieve it. I very much believe that if it is essential, you will make it. You will do all you can safely to achieve it.

When going out of your safe bubble, people will stare at you and try to work out what got you in a wheelchair. People will ask you because they somehow care or are plain curious as to your difference from them. Still, it will only highlight the differences between being able and not able. It might even make you angry and feel every negative emotion possible.

After months at home, I asked to do something I had done weekly before my injury: visit the supermarket. I wanted to compare the experience now with the experience then. For one, it took way longer. Inside, people would stare, and my husband had to adjust his wheelchair driving skills so that I could see the choices on offer. The biggest disappointment came at the checkout. He pushed me forward next to the checkout lady while he emptied the items of the cart. Then the checkout lady, completely ignoring me, turned her attention to my husband.

"Can she pay?"

Not only was I invisible, but she also made me incredibly sad. My husband did not miss a beat.

"If you want to get paid, you might want to ask her."

Horrible experience, and I never went to that supermarket again. Online supermarket shopping seemed a more inclusive experience. To paraphrase the words of Maya Angelou, I will forget what you said, I will forget what you did, but I will never forget how you made me feel.

The best experience was when we went to town to buy new shoes as my feet had swollen and I wanted a pair of shoes with secure fastenings. Not only did the salesperson get down to my level, but she took extra care in finding fashionable shoes that fitted my wishes. She made me feel as if I was the most important person at that moment. When it came to paying for the boots, she slid out a hidden shelf in the counter at my wheelchair height and placed a wireless card machine on there, which enabled me to pay for my purchase. I had a grin from ear to ear.

I am trying to convey that most people have no idea how to respond to you when they see you. Their response can be super helpful, like that of a loving parent or the opposite. You cannot change how other people act or react. You can only manage your response. You may well have to take steps to become less sensitive about comments made. That is a gradual process where you eventually accept that you look different, speak differently, and do things in a unique way. Today I give as good as I get.

Recently someone commented, "Shame you are in a wheelchair." The person was shocked at my response, "No, no, you are mistaken. That is my bike. It gets me from A to B. Without it, I would not be here." I wear colourful clothing and have my nails done because I want people to see me first, not me in the wheelchair. I leave my home, despite being in a wheelchair, and am no longer affected by their perception of me. I embody that the person I am is inside of me. I want to express who I am just like they do with their clothing, makeup, and language. If their perception of me is that of a lesser person disabled in a wheelchair, that does not automatically mean I have to conform to their image. I try to understand where they are coming from but always show them who I am and why I am there.

"You only get one shot at giving a first impression." My mother had drilled that into me. To her, it meant a clean dress, combed and plaited hair, clean hands, and a dazzling smile. Indeed, I would fail that with the little hair I had left, a crooked smile, twice my previous size, and in a wheelchair. How was I going to meet that challenge? Instead of looking immaculate, I translated it to mean being comfortable. No one could miss me. Armed with comfortable clothes, a bib, wipes in case I spilled something on my top, hair combed slick against my skull, brightly coloured nails, and a big smile on my face, I told everyone I had arrived. I would impersonate the diva who faced her public. What people thought of me was irrelevant. I was comfortable, and I was happy to be there and ready, flexible for anything.

There were plenty of embarrassing moments, but in the end, they forgave me since I was a person with a disability, and some allowances were made. One of those moments happened at a birthday party. I had told the hosts I would be attending in my electric powerchair, and they had made a special place for me, wide enough, at the first table. That also meant that if I needed to leave for the bathroom, I could, in principle, leave without disturbing anyone. It all went well at first.

Behind me, some two meters from where I was sitting, was another table, draped with a satin sheet upon which the cake took pride of place. Many people entered admiring the cake. Someone asked very nicely if I could sit a little more to the right of the table so that another person could fit in. I can do this, thinking I would slowly reverse the wheelchair, direct it to the right and sit back at the table. I started to do just that, then stopped to change directions when someone shouted, "STOP!" No idea of what was happening, I stopped and heard some noise behind me. After a few moments, the lady sitting next to me, who I had seen rushing out of her chair, said, "It's okay to go now, dear. You're free to get back."

When I was back at the table, she described how the satin sheet had got caught in my powerchair's wheel, without my knowledge. I was happily moving attached to the satin sheet upon which stood a fabulously artistic birthday cake. It had started to come to the edge of the table, and someone had been able to catch it just in time before it slid off. However, disaster averted. Not a moment where I faded in the background. Another embarrassing moment under my belt. So, if you must reverse, check what's behind you and make sure it's okay to drive forward. Thankfully, they saw the funny side.

There will be people who will avoid you. You may lose friends, which is heartbreaking. I went from having ten active friendships to having three. I took it very personally. After meditating on this, I discovered that those friendships had been me helping them when they went through a crisis. Once I could no longer do that physically, they disappeared from the horizon. The friendships that remained were far more joyous. They were the ones that accepted me for who I was and not for what I did. That is a great discovery to make. Just think of all that energy saved. Not only can you do what is essential, but you will also find time to spend with your most compatible friends. A handful these days, but I cherish them all. It is still a two-way conversation, and although I cannot go out with them, I am a good listener, which is valuable to them too.

16

MOVING FORWARD

In the midst of gathering darkness, light
becomes more evident.
— Bonnie Bostrom

I have always had a love affair with facts and
figures. I now use that interest to help monitor my
physical health. Doctors form their treatment plan
based on your feedback and data from blood tests
and scans. The medical professionals keep
checking your results to monitor the stability of
your health. You can do that too by giving your
body the nutrition it needs and investigating the
potential for exercise. You may be able to increase
your movement and fitness by gradually
exercising.

My way of doing something for my physical health involved weight training and stretches. Because going to the gym was impossible, I followed a little exercise routine of building up to one round of the garden in my wheelchair, reaching and moving things, stretching as much as possible. I practiced chair yoga and ultimately dreamed of going on a cycle ride with a custom-made hand bike. I would have included swimming as I loved to swim. However, the effort required in being dressed and undressed by a caregiver makes this exercise too exhausting to benefit me. Although the potential for leaving home is minimal, I found ways to learn and bring challenges into my life that would increase wellness in the future.

When you think you cannot change anything, you can try to investigate another area of your being in which you can make changes. Let us say I am too physically weak to push my wheelchair. I could leave it at that. If you do the same things, you will get the same outcome. I needed to increase the strength in my arms without gym equipment. Full bottles of water and tins of beans helped with weight training. Every day I would attempt to move in the wheelchair, and every day I would be grateful for something and some progress.

I believed I could, I persevered daily, and it created momentum. I got to know my wheelchair and its strengths and weaknesses, and all these actions made a difference. The accompanying mental work was never to give up. I could master this different body and work with it and not against it. Currently, I need to save for the next step, a hand bike for my wheelchair. Cycling in the countryside, feeling the wind in my hair, will provide a sense of freedom I so much enjoyed before my injury. Explore what, if anything, is possible to get the rush and excitement you experienced in the past. Keep looking, and you will find what suits you best now.

I spent much time alone with my thoughts. I decided to read the Bible, or as one of my sons calls it, the Book of Information Before Life Eternal. Spending more time on my spiritual pathway helped me better connect with my soul and my authentic self. It did not bring any immediate answers, but it was a companion and a teacher of patience. I identified most with the chapter on Job, who lost everything but not his faith, which strengthened me.

Whatever information you gather in your

journal, see what little changes you have made and how they affect the data you collect. How do you feel when you wake up? How is your appetite? What is ahead today in your schedule? What action can you take next, and how? What will you feel kind about and grateful for today?

Every action we take has a consequence. Of course, in most instances, our decisions will be positive, and the results positive too. Quite often, the little victories we celebrate because of the small steps we managed to take towards the future do not receive recognition. Every baby step towards your vision is worth celebrating. It brings you just that little closer to the ideal scenario of living your optimum life.

Personally, if I stay within the energy boundaries that my new body allows me, I can function at my optimum. That becomes my baseline. If my performance is lower than usual for any reason, I can analyze why. It is usually an infection my body is busy dealing with, or I have overstepped my energy allowance. Whatever the cause, I must respect it and adjust. Then, when I have recovered and am back at my optimum level, it allows me to prepare for the next challenge that presents itself. Be comfortable and at peace with

who you are. It will lead you confidently to the
authentic you.

I usually end my day by writing three things for
which I am grateful. If I am genuinely thankful for
all I have and take care of those things, it highlights
what increased my happiness that day and
establishes that, despite my struggles, I can be
content. I am grateful every day for something: the
sound of the rain, a pleasant family meal, and the
people that support me. Being grateful creates
positive feelings instead of dwelling on what did
not go well that day. It lifts energy and creative
thinking. Over the years, it astounds me that we
each use our twenty-four hours a day differently.
Sometimes in a more energy-intensive way, yet slow
and safe, you achieve the important things that
work towards your ideal day and purpose in life.

The medical profession will do all it can to
medically stabilize and replace the parts they can
restore to facilitate daily living. They do the best
they can with the resources and knowledge they
have, and you can too. Explore who you are, what
you want to do here, and take it to the next level.
All you see currently may be a barrier that has
shut down your hopes and dreams. If all you can
see is closed doors, go and find the window, create

a new outlook, and work out ways to safely get out there.

I remember an image my grandmother painted for me as a child. "When all is dark, and you feel overwhelmed, look out of your window, and search for the light. It may be the moon, it may be the sun, snow, or it may be the little flicker of a candle. Search for the light. Focus, and you will find that in every dark moment, there is a glimmer of light that signals hope."

17

PIERCING THE CHRYSALIS

You just need to accept the situation in which
you are and discover how beautiful it is.
— Beatrice 'Bebe' Vio

There is a moment in every health journey where
the balance shifts from your condition managing
your life to you managing your condition. It is a
subtle moment of grace. It is a moment of
acceptance as well as confidence in your new
abilities. Things still happen, but you know where
to look for imbalance and how to reverse that. My
baseline is a good indicator that works. Sticking to
how much I can comfortably do and planning
accordingly brings an absolute strength. It can be
tweaked so that if the weather is scorching, I will

need to hydrate more. Or if I have an infection, I need to do less, etc.

What is the plan when you feel unwell again, and how can you be prepared? I have developed unconscious signs that signal to my caregiver that all is not well. First, I stop talking (hard to imagine at the best of times). Next, I try to micromanage her. Bearing in mind, she does the same thing every day, there is no need for me to do that. My caregiver then is on the lookout for external signs.

As I have no feeling in parts of my body, I do not get the usual "pain signals," and she is my first responder. Once she identifies an issue, I try to rest more, be mindful of what is happening, and manage the situation. The next point of call is to contact my general practitioner, who, if necessary, will dispense extra medication and acts as the gatekeeper to specialized consultant care. It all takes a great deal of time and effort but having a list of contacts and knowing who to call brings absolute calm into a problematic situation. It takes the thinking out of the emergency and provides a clear action path where needed.

Your support team also will include people you trust and who do not mind if you become a moaning ninny and have them listen to your tyranny of woe. I am incredibly fortunate to have a long-suffering super patient partner and genuine friends who have stuck with me through this whole time. The support is mutual, but very mutual when I need help with any aspects of my health.

When you feel well enough to socialize, surround yourself with people who have the same interests and who like you. They will not see you as a disabled person but someone who tries to be authentic and has a good time. Time spent with a good friend, where mutual conversation happens, can be a balm to the soul.

My church community has been a great source of support too. They prayed for me, wrote me cards, and during the pandemic made sure to include me in their Zoom meetings enabling me to be a part of the church family again. That was a tremendous benefit during the COVID-19 restrictions.

Sometimes you need to be bold and ask for what you want. If I say, "I do not feel well," it might be construed as me complaining about nothing in particular. But if I say, "I have a pain in my liver, and I need you to check my blood to see what is going on," that gives a much better indication to my doctor how to move forward. When something different happens, and you are unclear what decision you need to make to move forward, at that moment, I invite you to get your journal. Revisit the progress you have made and the dreams your authentic self feels called to do. In time, with silence and reflection, you will begin to see a path clearing ahead.

Personally, my priorities are maintaining my meaningful relationships with my family. In practice, that means taking time to speak with them, support them, and encourage them when needed. My children know that I may not be there their entire lives, but they are confident they will have my love and attention during my lifetime.

There is time in my day to do some things I enjoy. I value doing what feeds my soul and makes me happy. As my children grew up, I found I had a great need to nurture my daily life, so I created a nano garden. It is accessible, small, and grows an abundance of fresh salad produce in the summer. It provides fresh food, space for me to breathe clean air, watch my plants grow, and enables me to exercise daily. Time spent in the garden is limited to ten minutes a day, but that still allows a task in the garden daily—a space I can cultivate fruits and vegetables. There is no better feeling or satisfaction than to pick a strawberry untouched by anyone and grown without chemicals as nature intended it.

There are things you can do by yourself in solitary moments, and there are moments that can be shared. I listen to audiobooks, music, and podcasts. I travel the world on my laptop and enjoy Netflix just like anyone else. Before the injury, I loved to cook and cooked often, but those tasks require too much energy now and present difficulties. However, I nurture my sourdough starter, Bread Pitt, feeding it twice weekly and, together with my husband, make a sourdough loaf once a week. Do you remember baking cookies with grandma and the feeling of closeness as you made something delicious to eat? My version is making sourdough bread with my husband. It envelops me in the same feelings of closeness I had with grandma in my childhood.

In the past, I did all sorts of fibre crafts, from spinning fleeces into yarn, dying the yarn into all kinds of colours, and knitting and weaving cloth for my handmade wardrobe. Everyone will have a favourite activity or many of them. Find your passion and do those activities as much as possible. Play, and enjoy that time of creation.

Knowing what you are capable of, and having a direction to pursue, enables you to declutter your possessions and say goodbye to those things that remind you too much of the past. My weaving loom found a new home with a new weaver. I donated all my dye books to a new up-and-coming dyer. Spreading the joy and memory of the craft I had experienced made me happy.

Do not dwell too long on the things you can no longer do but give energy to those activities within your capability. Do more of what you can do, bearing in mind that just because you can do it does not mean you have to do it. Yes, with some help I can make a birthday cake. But I do not have the time or energy to make it as well as spend time with my beloved friend. I prefer to get someone else to make the cake and see the joy in her face when the cake is put in front of her. We can then both enjoy the birthday moment. That exhausts me, but I get the most reward from the moment without risking immediate exhaustion.

Before my injury, I did too much, feared too much, and had truly little time to devote to self-care. My relationships, including my relationship with God, suffered as a result. With hindsight, I could even go as far as to say that what happened, happened to redress the balance in my life. From that moment on, I have gradually started to emerge out of it better and better. Broken in parts, yet whole as a result.

The butterfly shows us a beautiful symmetrical pattern on its wings as it flies in the fields, touching the centre of many flowers and weeds. A rosebud, similarly, is not that interesting to look at closed. But when it trusts the light, the rain, and the care it receives, it gradually opens. It reveals a lovely shaped bloom, possible overpowering scent, and its beauty all at once. It may only last for a short, intense time, but it reached its potential as it was meant to. We can choose to see rosebushes as bushes with thorns, or we can marvel at the fact that bushes with thorns ultimately provide the gift of a rose.

I compare the process of becoming myself to that of the caterpillar becoming a butterfly. The caterpillar spends some time in its chrysalis hidden from the world before emerging as a butterfly. It spreads its wings, flies, enjoying every moment. The butterfly flies from flower to flower, enjoying the nectar. Its purpose will be to lay its eggs somewhere safe before it dies, often within a short time span. Its life may seem traumatic and brief, and yet it fulfils its purpose. Without being in my cocoon, I would never have had the experience to enable me to write this book for you.

My wish is to help others facing the dreadful moment in which they believe their life dissolves without joy.

In hindsight, I can be thankful for coming through all those awful experiences, climbing that mountain, crawling up the hill to emerge at the top. It made it possible for me to enjoy the view and be closer to God and the universe He created.

His creation is beautiful and complicated. Many things happen in His timing, not yours or mine. All the experiences and knowledge gained through various jobs and complicated relationships prepared me for dealing with an impossible reality. I thought of having my dreams stolen and all joy robbed. If I had believed that I was possible, and nothing is impossible, my painful journey would have been less painful.

> Your path led through the sea, your way through the mighty waters, though your footprints were not seen.
> — Psalm 77, Verse 19

I am carried in the arms of my God to the other side of the beach. I feel humbled that the Shepherd left His ninety-nine sheep to come and find me to tend to me.[1] I am unable to walk, yet He carries me. When I was lost, I listened for the knocking of His shepherd's crook against the mountain wall. Arriving at the top of the mountain, I have a spectacular view, fresh air, and sunshine.

18

EMERGING

Stand in the ashes of the barn burned down, pointing to the moon. One half in suffering and one half in hope.
— Lauralee Farrer

In Taekwondo, the first position is called Joon Bi, the ready stance. Writing this book is a way for me to be with you while facing your dark moment of the soul and help you get into your "ready stance." Being in your Joon Bi stance of strength and living in the moment will provide stability. You may feel you are alone in your room with no idea how to move or move forward. I am here to let you know that you have everything you need to create a life worth living that will serve you and others.

When we suffer an injury, we suffer in all areas of our being. That means mentally, emotionally, and spiritually as well as physically. Our families and relationships suffer too, and without adapting to our new way of being in the world, broken but whole, we remain vulnerable. We can take action to create an imaginary safe bubble around ourselves to minimise and absorb any impacts we could experience without that bubble.

A support team will give you confidence when life gets out of balance and your health demands immediate attention. Your support team can be there to get help as quickly and effectively as possible, so you have the time and opportunity to have moments and adventures that feed you. With a framework surrounding you, you will have the foundations to rebuild your reality one day at a time.

Take time to clarify what you are striving for and why you are doing what you do. Let your support team know what is changing and not changing so that you will know how to move forward into the future. Think about how you are communicating this process to your support team and accepting feedback. Have real conversations about changes you need to make and get feedback from your support team on how you are going forward and what that means for them. Some steps will take you forward, and some will not.

You could be on the floor, depleted, discouraged, and bewildered, wondering what could have gone worse. It is not only about your disability; it's about focusing on and reframing the future. If you need a coach or a therapist to get that objective view, seek that help. Options are available online.

Tell yourself, nothing is impossible because I am possible. When things are tough, show up, keep going, and carry on. The other option, giving in and doing nothing, is not known to lead to getting through it.

In this personal account, I used the lifecycle of the butterfly as a metaphor. It represents the transformation that happens on all levels of being as a result of significant trauma. The caterpillar evolves, not once, but twice, first from a larva to a caterpillar, and then into a beautiful butterfly. If there is one thing we can learn from the humble caterpillar, it's that change is possible.

The chrysalis is one of the most enduring symbols in the natural world. It is the place of transformation. Within it, the body that once served its purpose is discarded in favour of another. The former body is broken, and something very different will emerge. The new body is for something different. The transformation begins with a horrifying process. But this process contains everything needed to create the butterfly. Everything about the creature changes during this process - the way it looks, moves, senses, and functions. Yet not everything is broken. The true essence of the creature remains - its authentic self, which is not limited to the confines of its metamorphosed body.

During the process of healing physically and transforming our bodies and minds, we have the ability to find our authentic selves; our 'why' for existing, as well as a way to express our unique contribution in this world. We have different challenges, different priorities, and different abilities. Having a disability does not define who you are, but may limit or challenge the way you express who you are in this world. We may no longer be completely independent, but with the support of carefully chosen and significant others, we can find our way to express our authenticity and find our voice in the world.

It is time to create your future. Take the reboot moment, pick yourself up, humble yourself. We all need to learn something new and trust people differently. Give people the freedom to say thank you and leave. Everything is working out correctly. We do not get to where we are without accidents. There is something that led us up to now. We always get the results for which we planted the seeds. Reflect on what got you here, how and why it happened. Now you can know that what you do matters and do what matters to you most. Make the right decisions and sow new seeds.

Everything is the way it should be. You can create a future to ensure you get what you want. Make conscious decisions on what you want and do not want from now on. Take action to get out of where you are. Baby steps will do, one virtual foot in front of the other. You got this.

Life is a continuous trail of moments. Instead of planning what you want to do in ten years, you will be stable and ready for the next moment. Keep your vision board in mind. You will be secure in your authentic self with a clearer vision of the direction you are going in. Expect the unexpected. You will be protected with the armour of God. He is at your every side and will provide stability, protection, and direction.

However the traumatic event arrived in your life, however painful and impossible the future looks, try and find the seed within you that is waiting to germinate and find its unique expression in the world around you. Let my story of transformation through carefully structured baby steps, underpinned by a steely determination, encourage you to break through your chrysalis. Emerge, spread your wings, and take flight as a stronger, more beautiful expression of your true self.

ACKNOWLEDGEMENTS

My eternal thanks go to my family and friends who walked beside me. To Aleathea Dupree for holding my hand throughout the writing of this book and working towards publishing it.

Thank you to Mark, Neil, David, and all the medical staff for persevering in their quest to find out the reason my body was malfunctioning.

Thanks to my support network and Pauline for never failing to encourage me from day to day and for handling my daily health and care needs. Without your support, I would be less able to be who I have become.

A special thank you to my husband, who has never failed to believe in me. He has always been my rock, my East to West.

And a special thank you for prayers answered.

NOTES

Preface

1. Hits (or knocked) for six means to shock, overwhelm, or completely devastate someone, especially suddenly. Primarily heard in the United Kingdom and Australia.

Introduction

1. Haidt, Jonathan. *The Happiness Hypothesis: Putting Ancient Wisdom to the Test of Modern Science*. London: Arrow Books, 2006.

1. The Main Event

1. A tram is a public transport vehicle, usually powered by electricity from wires above it, which travels along rails laid in the surface of a street. Also known in some places as a streetcar or trolley.
2. A lesion is an area in an organ or tissue which has suffered damage through injury or disease.
3. A registrar in the United Kingdom is a hospital ward's senior doctor and is usually contactable on site, while the senior consultant (or specialist) attends ward rounds and meetings at specific times.

2. Strengthening the Things Which Remain

1. A cottage hospital is a smaller hospital closer to your place of residence. It is a place where local familiar people can visit you or where they hold you while they decide what the next medical action is.

3. The Needle in the Haystack

1. *Futurama* is an American animated science fiction television series created by Matt Groening.

17. Piercing the Chrysalis

1. The Parable of the Lost Sheep is one of the parables of Jesus. It is about a shepherd who leaves his flock of ninety-nine sheep in order to find the one which is lost. It appears in the Gospels of Matthew (Matthew 18:12–14) and Luke (Luke 15:3–7).

RESOURCES

In this section, I have included a list of books, websites, and other resources that have helped me in my journey. I trust this information will also be helpful in yours.

Apps

Calm, Guided Meditation & Sleep

Articles

Helgeson, Vicki S., Kerry A. Reynolds, and Patricia L. Tomich. "A Meta-Analytic Review of Benefit Finding and Growth." *Journal of Consulting and*

Clinical Psychology 74, no. 5 (2006): 797–816. https://doi.org/10.1037/0022-006x.74.5.797.

Books

Follow Your North Star by Martha Beck

Gratefulness, The Heart of Prayer: An Approach to Life in Fullness by David Steindl-Rast

The Happiness Hypothesis: Putting Ancient Wisdom and Philosophy to the Test of Modern Science by Jonathan Haidt

Life Without Limits: Inspiration for a Ridiculously Good Life by Nick Vujicic

The Lord of the Rings by J.R.R. Tolkien

Mary Poppins by P. L. Travers

The Medical Science of House, M.D. by Andrew Holtz

The Power of Now by Eckhart Tolle

Other

Thunderbirds. (Television Series) ATV Midlands, September 30, 1965.

'Allo 'Allo! (Television Series) BBC One, December 30, 1982.

Websites

Go Gently with Michael Nobbs. www.gogently.co

Jacquie Lawson (Artist), Animated Ecards. www.jacquielawson.com

Monk Manual (Journal), A Daily System for Being and Doing. www.monkmanual.com

SendOutCards, Online Greeting Card System. www.sendoutcards.com

Touchnote, Personalized Cards and Photo Gifts. www.touchnote.com

YouTube

Calm (Channel), 10 Minutes of Mindfulness. www.youtube.com/c/calm

DDP Yoga. (Video) "Never, Ever Give Up. Arthur's Inspirational Transformation!" April 30, 2012.

Wheels2Walking with Richard Corbett Podcast (Channel)

WheelsNoHeels with Gem Hubbard. (Channel) www.youtube.com/c/wheelsnoheels

Yoga Nidra Guide. (Channel) www.youtube.com/user/yoganidraguide

Yoga Nidra with Lizzy Hill. (Channel) www.youtube.com/c/LizzyHill22

ABOUT THE AUTHOR

Josephine is the mother of four and married to her silent partner, who chooses to remain anonymous. When she is not wheeling around town on her "bicycle," she can be found tilting perspectives about being differently able, being authentic, and living an optimal life despite disability.

www.josephinemariposa.com

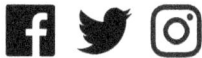